The
Serotonin-Insulin
Connection

The Link to Achieving Extraordinary
Physical and Mental Health

THE BRAIN CHEMISTRY SOLUTION

Control Cravings and Overcome Addictions
The Link Between Mental Health and Our Nutrition
Alleviate Depression and Anxiety
Why Cholesterol is Vital to Longevity
Reduce Risks for Alzheimer's
Lose Body Fat Without Going Hungry
Prevent and Reverse Common Diseases
Look and Feel Years Younger

Phoenix Gilman

G&G PUBLISHING

The Serotonin-Insulin Connection
Copyright © 2021 Phoenix Gilman
ISBN 13: 978-0-578-95536-0

* Previously titled: Diet Failure the Naked Truth / Three previous editions 2012 - 2016

PUBLISHER: G&G Publishing
COPY EDITOR: Martha Sigwart
GRAPHIC DESIGN: Billy Ciampo & Phoenix Gilman
PHOTOGRAPHY: Phoenix (back cover, pages 48, 52, 118, 132, 143, 150, 161, 162, 194, 198, 206, 214, 215)

This book is dedicated to
my father, mother and grandmother,
and to my loyal, loving friends,
who have always been there for me,
Peggy, Billy, Janene and Evelyn.

To my husband, Christopher,
you are my everything!
I am grateful for the life, and love, we share.

—Phoenix

"How do I tell you, where do I begin?
How do you thank someone for giving them the gift of hope—and life?
You truly are a blessing in this world, Phoenix!"

— Karla Jo Wood

"What you have done in this book is probably more powerful than you know and will
ultimately help more people than you can possibly imagine.
Congratulations! Life's purpose fulfilled!"

— Kelly Davis, Mother, Business Executive

"I know your life's work can sometimes feel more like a job than a mission,
but I want you to know your work is so important. You are really changing lives.
Because of you, my grandchildren will never struggle with their weight, mood, or energy,
and they will live much healthier. That type of generational influence is so powerful.
You will be part of my family far beyond even when I'm gone.
What I have learned from you will transcend anything I ever expected.
Thank you! And I truly love you for who you are—and what you represent."

— Raquel Riffas, Mother, Radiologic Technologist, Vascular Intervention

With Gratitude

Long ago, I discovered the indescribable bond that is shared with a true friend. For me, it is those special few who come into your life and completely accept you for who you are, without ever feeling the need to change you, judge you, or treat you less than. They don't pretend to have your back—only to find out that they are the ones you need protection from. Instead, they support you. Believe in you. Respect you. They love you unconditionally. All without ever betraying that sacred bond of friendship. This, however, is sadly very rare. I, therefore, feel extraordinarily blessed to have such wonderful friends throughout my life. To those who have shared their lives with me so selflessly, I am eternally grateful. To those who have helped and encouraged me along this venture, thank you.

To my father, Frank Gilman, thank you for your many sacrifices so that your children could have a better life. Though you gave to us above and beyond, I've come to appreciate most, all those not-so-little things we often take for granted, i.e., feeling safe and secure, clean clothes, a warm bed, never knowing hunger, regular medical/dental checkups, access to unlimited athletic opportunities, and a good education. And while I believe our character evolves as we grow, you gave me a strong foundation in which to grow from. Through the many years since then, thank you for always being there for me, drying my tears, loving me, and most of all, for finally coming to understand that all I really want from you is to be heard. And, though, you don't always understand or agree, thank you for respecting my free-spirit and desperate need to live a life that is true. Your love for me is such a blessing. <u>**UPDATE**</u>: No words can convey how grateful I am that you believed enough in my work that you wanted to write Oprah. Because of that letter, her staff has since requested a copy of my book. After nearly nine years of trying to get through her doors, it was the unwavering love of you, my father, that has finally caught their attention. I'm so thankful for you, in so many ways. I love and miss you!

Peggy Collins, who has since passed on, there is not a single day that goes by that I don't miss you. Since the day I first met you at merely 18, and you, stunning at 64, you showed me nothing but respect, kindness, and a love I had never before known. You were far more than my best friend, you were the mother I never had. You loved me completely. Without conditions. You guided me. Cared for me. Nurtured me. You took such pride in who I was as a person, as a young lady. I love and miss you beyond measure!

Billy Ciampo, we're far more than best of friends, we are family. You love me like I'm your own. You care for me. You respect my spirited nature. You watch out for me, as I do likewise for you. You're one of my greatest blessings. Thank you, as well, for giving so much of your personal time and artistic talents to help me bring to life my endless creative visions over the years, particularly my books. (I know it wasn't easy, but thank you for letting go and allowing me to create.) I love you and I am forever grateful for our friendship.

My grandmother, Harriet Vander Molen-Gilman, who has also passed on, you were an incredible woman, a woman so far ahead of your time. Thank you for showing me what living a healthy lifestyle is all about. Thank you for showing me that life is meant to be lived to the absolute fullest, regardless of age. Thank you for sharing such a loving, adventurous relationship with me. I love and miss you every single day!

My mother, Barbara Holcombe-Gilman, though you were, regrettably, taken from me at such a young age, I'm so thankful that many years later, I was able to spend time with you and get to know you, not only as my biological mother, but also as a friend, and as a loving, compassionate human being. You are an amazingly kind, caring, funny, and sensitive soul. Your love, your sincere sense of pride in me, is truly overwhelming. I love you and miss our days shared.

Janene Bogardus, my wonderful, ever-so-protective friend of over 40 years, I cherish you. Our friendship, our love for one another, is one of the purest bonds of all. No matter my joy, no matter my sorrow, you have always been there for me. I love you!

Evelyn and Julius Shapiro, I'm sincerely touched by your support, love, and belief in me and my work. Thank you for all that you so selflessly give me. I am honored to be your friend. I love and miss you!

Michael Murray, ND, celebrated naturopathic doctor, speaker, and best-selling author, thank you for taking the time to read my manuscript—and being willing to offer such a generous quote. Your continued, and encouraging support, is appreciated more than I can say.

Ken Buckner, Centers for Disease Control, your authenticated, relentless support means the world to me. I am continually grateful for all that you've done to so passionately share my work with others. You are, equally, an exceptional example of one who realized what can be achieved by simply following the truth I've outlined within this book. After all, as you well know, all things are possible.

Diana Schwarzbein, MD, leading endocrinologist, speaker, and best-selling author, thank you for taking the time to meet with me. Thank you for sharing my passion and encouraging my efforts. Your support was enormously flattering.

Stephen Scheinberg, PhD, MD, one of my most loyal, successful clients, I am so proud of all the changes you've made. I'm equally grateful for your endless support in endorsing my work.

Bruce Wiseman, U.S. President of Citizens Commissions for Human Rights, your efforts to make a difference is truly inspiring. As such, I'm honored that you have allowed me to share my research with your worldwide organization. Thank you, as well, for so graciously endorsing my work.

C.J. Yesson, thank you for your friendship and powerful, thought-provoking quote.

Ingrid Newkirk, PETA co-founder/president, thank you for all that you do to protect—and save the lives of animals! Your willingness to advocate my work is also greatly appreciated.

To my many faithful clients, customers, friends, and family, thank you for making the commitment to living a healthier lifestyle—and for helping me spread this amazing message of truth.

To my various chemists/formulators, thank you for allowing me to expect nothing, but perfection.

To those who have believed enough in my work to donate/sponsor my efforts, there are no words.

To those Body by Phoenix clients who shared so beautifully in our partnership, thank you for allowing me the opportunity to change your life in so many exciting ways. Such inspiration! I am grateful.

To the Infinite Intelligence that has blessed, inspired, and guided me throughout my life—and particularly this journey—I am eternally grateful for your quiet, yet constant presence in my life.

To the many dogs I've been fortunate enough to rescue, and love, I am eternally grateful. To those loyal companions who have sadly passed on, I miss your sweet, loving, and ever-protective souls. There is no greater, no purer love than that which I shared with each of you. Your selfless, oh, so innocent souls reminded me each and everyday to live in the moment; moreover, that nothing else really matters in this life except to give love—and be loved. Oooh, how I love and miss each and every one of you!

"Phoenix delivers a passionate, well-written blueprint for success in
weight loss and other challenges linked to low serotonin levels,
including sugar cravings, depression and insomnia."

— Michael T. Murray, ND, Co-Author, *Encyclopedia of Natural Medicine*

"Phoenix has provided us with the truth and nothing, but the truth.
Thus, the masses can take control and begin to be healthy once again.
Phoenix has given the most precious gift that anyone could ever ask for: 'The Fountain of Youth.'
All we have to do is take the initial step to drink from it—and the results are unlimited."

— Ken Buckner, Centers for Disease Control

"Phoenix explains, in explicit yet simple detail, the underlying cause of cravings,
carb addictions, even ADD, depression, and heart disease. Serotonin is truly the crucial
link to overcome obesity—and numerous other health issues. As a physician, scientist,
and formerly overweight person, I recommend everyone read this book, especially parents.
It will change, if not save, your life and the lives of your children."

— Stephen Scheinberg, PhD, MD

"Phoenix is one of the most amazing people I have ever come across in the world of diet and
health. Her passionate cry for sanity in such an insane world chock full of so-called experts and
pundits stands out above the rest. Prepare to be challenged, and then changed forever, after reading her book. Thank you, Phoenix, for staying true to the cause you believe in so strongly.
I encourage you to keep doing what you're doing for many more years to come!"

— Jimmy Moore, Weight Loss Blogger, Author
Livin' La Vida Low Carb

"Phoenix has given all of us a tremendous gift in this well researched and
comprehensive book about diet failure. Our struggle for effective and healthy weight
loss is universal. In all my years of radio and numerous interviews, this book shares
crucial information and an understanding for weight loss success that I have
never heard from anyone else. What a gift!"

— Brad Walton / The Brad Walton Show – WCCO – CBS Radio

"You have touched me in more ways than you will ever know! You are a great person that truly cares for what you believe in. I will always bet on you to win the race anytime!"

— Angela L. Smith

"You did for me what physicians, naturopaths, chiropractors, gastroenterologists, and others could not. I feel so much better. My health is truly transformed. So thankful!"

— Kim Matthews

"Phoenix, you are my golden ticket to better health and a leaner body!! I am so thankful for finding you, your book, and your work. I have never felt better in all my life! I will be forever grateful!!!"

— Jenny Eberhard

"People must wake up to the consequences of treating their bodies—and animals—badly. This book contributes to this wake-up call."

— Ingrid Newkirk, PETA Co-Founder/President

"I don't know how to ever thank you, but I hope you know that you have done good in the world. Like the story of the starfish, if it is only one you save,it means a lot to that one. Me."

— Sharon S, Sales Manager

"Phoenix is a wise woman who has taken it upon herself to stand in the darkness holding the candle of truth for us to see. What she advises is factual, reasonable, and more importantly, doable. There is nothing in her book that is beyond grasp for a lifetime. I owe this woman my life."

— Gerry Hillburn, Wife, Mother, Caregiver

CONTENTS

With Gratitude vii

Disclaimer. xv

Introduction: *Managing Expectations*. xvii

PART 1

The Serotonin-Insulin Connection Revealed

1 Why 98% of All Diets Fail 5
The missing link needed to overcome obesity

2 Serotonin: An Extraordinary Brain Chemical 9
A carb addict you are not

3 Oh, the Many Diets We've Fallen Prey To 19
From starvation to the low fat myth

4 This is NOT a Diet 27

5 Health Conditions Associated with Low Serotonin 31
Obesity, diabetes, alcoholism, insomnia, depression, anxiety, etc.

6 How to Naturally Boost Serotonin 33
All natural supplement, no drugs needed

7 The Remarkable Health Benefits of 5-HTP 37

8 Unheard of, but Why? 43

9 Storing Body Fat 49
One of insulin's many roles

10 Type 2 Diabetes Running Rampant 53
Self-induced, yet so easy to reverse

11 Sugar & Its Highly Addictive Nature 57
Stronger than any street drug

12 The Many Faces of Sugar 61

13 WARNING: High-Fructose Corn Syrup 63

14 Aspartame—A DEADLY TOXIN 67
Making us fat, depressed & deathly ill

15 Obesity, an Alarming Epidemic 73

16 Fat Cells Gettin' Fatter. 77

17 All Stimulants Become Depressants 81
"Got coffee?"

18 Direct Link Between Mental Health & Our Nutrition. 85
You are what you eat; physically & mentally

19 Insulin & How It Affects Cholesterol. 103
Avoid junk carbs, instead, eat healthy fat & cholesterol

20 Insulin & How It Affects Blood Pressure 109

21 Eating Healthy Without Ever Feeling Deprived. 113

22 Marketing Scams That Are Making Us Fatter & Sicker Than Ever. 119

23 From Petting Zoo to Dinner Table 127
When did it go so terribly wrong?

24 Exercise, Nutrition & Hormones 133
A tricky balance to achieve optimum health

25 Genes. 145
Use 'em or abuse 'em

26 Expect More from Yourself. 151
Self-care is a must

27 "Got Abs?" 163
One of the biggest weight loss myths

28 Pharmaceutical Drugs & Their Side Effects. 165
Weight gain, depression, heart failure, new disease, even death

PART II

Carbohydrates & the Glycemic Index

28 What is a Carb? 183

30 Good Carb? Bad Carb?. 185
    Which is it?

31 Crucial Carbohydrate Facts 191

32 My Personal Meals that Will Help You
    Lose body fat, improve lipids, alleviate depression, increase energy—and more 195

33 How to Read a Nutrition Facts Label 199
    Don't be fooled. Know what you're eating.

34 Summary of Health Tips 207
    That will help you achieve optimum health

PART III

In Closing

Body by Phoenix Client Testimonials. 210

Research/References 212

In Loving Memory 214

Author 215

"As a consumer, this book is, at minimum, enlightening, but more so alarming. As a businessman, I discovered a whole world of underexposed, unethical possibilities. As a human being, Phoenix created new hope for a better life. More than a case study of the diet question, this book is an extensive discovery of everything that is good for you. Well worth reading. Well worth memorizing."

— C.J. Yesson, Retired Life Insurance CEO, Investment Banker

"This book is a comprehensive and insightful analysis of diets, why so many fail, and what it takes to succeed. Phoenix shows the reader the critical role of insulin in fat storage and serotonin in our mental life, the two main ingredients for successful dieting. A necessary read for anyone interested in leading a healthier and happier life."

— Dr. Jay D. Glass, PhD (Neuroscience & Psychology), Author

"A very provocative book. The science is thoroughly researched and well-documented. And if one follows Phoenix's advice, amazing, life-altering results will no doubt follow. A truly worthwhile guide to healthy living."

— Rex A. Licklider, Vice Chairman/CEO, The Sports Club Company

Phoenix has done the research and knows what it takes to get you where you need to be. She speaks from her heart—and with more compassion than anyone I know."

—Tammy Boyd, Wife, Mother, Grandmother

"Phoenix shines the light of truth on how today's seemingly endless new array of psychiatric 'diseases' have underlying physical causes, which are best addressed by proper nutrition and healthcare—not the growing panoply of toxic psychiatric drugs. This book, particularly the 'Pharmaceutical Drugs and Their Side Effects' chapter, provides extremely important information for today's health conscious consumer."

— Bruce Wiseman, U.S. President, Citizens Commission on Human Rights

DISCLAIMER

No particular product that is formulated and/or owned by the author is being promoted, sold, or endorsed in this book. It is, instead, about individual herbs/extracts/amino acids/vitamins/minerals, etc. Any references made by the author, including, but not limited to R&D (Research & Development), products, supplements, testing stages, clients, client's results, etc., were done entirely for the purpose of conveying a point of expertise. Any principles and/or health benefits discussed can be easily achieved with similar products. This book's sole purpose is to educate the consumer as to the research within. And, to reiterate, this book is not intended to diagnose, treat, cure, or prevent any illness. This book is the sole opinion of Phoenix Gilman, the author. It was written merely to inform the reader. It is not intended as medical advice. It should not be used to replace any medical care or any therapeutic program recommended by a medical doctor. The author (and publisher) disclaim any and all liability arising directly or indirectly from the use of the information contained within this book.

"I have a very strong and developed 'truth meter' and it was screaming that you were an authentic messenger of the truth in the crazy, deceptive, confusing, demoralizing world of food addiction and weight loss. Phoenix, you have impacted my life like a lighthouse beacon shining in utter darkness."

— Mary Imes, MS, Speech Pathologist

"Path to wellness you strive to do your best. Along the way you meet someone like Phoenix that makes you think and find the true self you've been hiding. She offers support, friendship and a gentleness that brings clarity, self-respect to light. I am amazed at the success of it all. Thank you for helping me find me."

— Sue Schneider

"Phoenix, in body, heart, and soul, is like a perfect diamond, brilliant and multi-faceted. She exquisitely radiates crystal clear nutritional truths. Her cutting-edge 'control the cravings' research fearlessly exposes dieting flaws and myths. Her uniquely courageous self-disclosure energizes, implores, and motivates. She lovingly serves up practical and doable success strategies unparalleled by others in the weight loss world."

— Judy Krings, PhD, Clinical Psychologist, Personal Coach

"Phoenix deserves to be heralded as a researcher and author who could reverse our nation's obesity epidemic—both childhood and adult—one previously failed dieter at a time. It will remain one of the most important books on the subject of cravings, food addiction, and permanent weight loss you will ever read and re-read, and then you, too, will thank Phoenix for her invaluable work."

— Larry W., Founder, Recovery Talk Network

"You care more about others, even strangers, and getting this extraordinary information and message out, than being a profit hungry fiction writer. It is amazing to go through life, as you have experienced, and still have a great love for people. There is no word in any language to describe the extraordinary person you really are. This is what attracts me to the TRUTHFULNESS of your book. You are no fool and you are not trying to fool anyone. You have stripped yourself bare and exposed what truly matters in your heart and you have nothing to hide. You are not in it for selfish gain! That kind of honesty is very rare, very very rare!"

— A. Hayes

INTRODUCTION
Managing Expectations

I've written this book with the sincerest desire to help others understand why 98% of all diets fail—and equally why depression, anxiety, ADD, diabetes, hypertension, even heart disease—are so disturbingly prevalent. This breakthrough information is based on proven clinical research, not diet or marketing hype. To ensure you get the utmost from the information presented, I respectfully ask that you please first carefully read the following:

1) This is not a diet or a quick fix. I am not promising, "Lose 30 pounds in 30 days!" My suggested lifestyle program is, though, about how to live a much *healthier lifestyle*. So please, don't stress over losing the excess weight. It will come. I promise you. Focus instead on healing your body and mind. Just remember, it took a lifetime to damage your body. It will equally take time to reverse the damage. It will also require effort and consistency to achieve your various goals. You must be willing to do what it takes.

2) I wrote my book in a Q&A format, as it best reflected the actual dialogue exchanged between me and my clients, and even total strangers simply seeking advice on any given day. It was also crucial that I represent the average consumer, that I directly voice their viewpoints, concerns, and countless frustrations. Some questions may seem trivial to one, but extremely helpful to another. In addition, I needed to challenge my own viewpoints, play the devil's advocate, so to speak.

3) Based on the far too confusing information provided by the AMA, FDA, and our very own doctors, I felt it was necessary to address all such issues in an easy-to-comprehend and personal tone, minus the usual over-the-top medical jargon that tends to confuse people even more. Nonetheless, this information is still very serious—and life-saving.

4) I was intentionally repetitive, because it often requires saying something repeatedly, and in various ways, before someone can grasp certain information in its entirety.

5) To further assist you in reaching your goals, please read cover to cover. Also, stop and ask yourself how the information relates to you and yours. Underscore those points of interest. It's essential that you then apply the knowledge in your daily life. Review this book often. Once you get it, your life will forever be changed.

6) This is *not* about perfection. Just eat according to your goals.

7) You'll lose inches before you actually lose a lot of weight. So please don't judge your success by the scale, as it's not an accurate assessment. Instead, measure your waist (an inch above the belly button), and insulin gauge (widest girth of the stomach/right in front of the belly button). Because this is the most harmful weight we carry, this is what you want to focus on. Track these two measurements.

8) Throughout the book, I use both the terms "weight loss" and "fat loss." My focus, though, is always about losing excess body fat. Another good reason to avoid the scale, as it's not so much about a number, as it is about losing excess body fat, while gaining lean muscle.

9) This book will give you the solution, as to why diets most often fail. I will equally teach you how to live free of so-called mental health issues, i.e., depression, anxiety, panic attacks, etc. FACT: Our nutrition plays a critical role in our mental health. Yet no one, *and I mean no one*, is talking about this. I will teach you how to mitigate your addictions/cravings for carbs/sugar, alcohol, nicotine and caffeine—and safely alleviate your depression, anxiety, insomnia, and so much more.

10) To those who have asked, *"Who are you? Are you a doctor? What is your degree?"*
I modestly reply: I'm a woman who seeks the truth. Always have. Always will. I'm a woman who wants to make a difference. I want to teach others how to help save their own lives by living a healthy lifestyle. I'm a woman who, after 20 plus years of being involved in various degrees of health and wellness, was fed up with the misinformation and marketing scams running rampant within the diet, food, and pharmaceutical industries—deceit that borders on criminal, and, at bare minimum, makes Americans fat, depressed, and sicker than ever.

I freely admit I'm not a doctor; nor do I need to be. This also means I'm not motivated by drug sales. I don't have a college degree; nor is it obligatory. (Though I earned a full four year scholarship at MI State based on my academics.) Equally, my alleged expertise doesn't come simply from "reading" medical journals or allowing some professor to tell me what is true. My expertise comes, instead, from an insatiable desire to educate myself; spending years diligently researching neurochemistry and nearly every aspect of nutrition. But that wasn't enough. I needed to actually test the many remarkable claims. So I developed various supplements, based on the research. What I witnessed throughout the four years of R&D with my company's products, is what prompted me to write my books. I knew, *without a doubt,* that all the clinical studies that I had read, all the amazing research that I had studied for years, was in fact, true.

11) I humbly exposed myself throughout the book, as it was important that the reader know I'm not just a researcher, but have actually experienced most of what I speak of, both good and bad. As such, the book will be at one moment serious and scientific, the next provocative, challenging, and in your face, to then playful and sexually frank. The next second it may make you cry, get angry, or dare you to rethink your life. All such honest emotions expressed will hopefully help keep the reader's attention from cover to cover. My motive? I want to force you, the reader, to think, to feel, to fight for your rights, to reach outside yourself, and to live a healthier, more compassionate life. For those who may be offended by my candor, language used, or choice of images, please don't be. The information I needed to share, goes far beyond the science.

Furthermore, I'm hoping that by sharing so much of my very private world, it will give you a better idea of who I am as a human being, as a woman with that certain edge, more so, as a compassionate, sensitive, strong-willed individual, so that, hopefully, in some small way, it will encourage you to live a happier, fuller, more determined life, one that is true to you, and those you care for. To also help you find the emotional, mental, and physical strength when you feel less than. And, to hopefully inspire you to discover your own unique passion and go after it. Because you see, throughout my life I have endured many struggles and heartaches. But I'm also a survivor. I believe in myself. I've never allowed others to drag me down or abuse me, be it verbally, mentally or physically. And, I never give up. Ever. All things are possible, if you believe in yourself and persevere.

12) This book is a revised edition of my three previous books titled, *Diet Failure the Naked Truth.* Considering my research can potentially help millions, especially since COVID, I felt it was important to launch a 4th and final edition, but with a new title, the latest research, medical updates, etc. (This is also why there are images of Billy and I at various ages.)

If you want to learn about my research that I titled, *The Serotonin-Insulin Connection*, please read this book from cover to cover.

More importantly, if you want to learn how you can safely, and effectively, mitigate addictions for carbs/sugar, alcohol, nicotine and caffeine, stop a transfer of addictions, alleviate mood swings, depression, anxiety, panic attacks, ADD/ADHD, PMS, and insomnia, reverse obesity, type 2 diabetes, osteoporosis, eliminate "high cholesterol" concerns, reduce excess body fat and triglycerides, while increasing HDL, lower your risks for heart disease, certain cancers (especially colon cancer) and dementia, stabilize blood pressure, add quality years to your life, while taking 10-20 years off your looks (no facelift needed), increase your energy exponentially, and improve your overall health in so many rewarding ways, all without drugs, and in record time, please read this book from cover to cover— and then implement what you've learned. It is truly life-changing/life-saving.

Finally, my intentions with this book are pure and simple: To educate. To inspire. To empower, especially women. To give hope. To make a difference. I sincerely hope it helps you live a much longer, happier, and healthier life.

Wishing you the greatest of success in health, in love, in life.

Phoenix

Entrepreneur, Researcher, Product Developer, Self-Published Author
Weight Loss/Anti-Aging Expert, Personal Trainer, Sports Nutritionist
Business Owner, Consumer Activist, Motivational Speaker

Johns Hopkins researchers looked at brain scans and
discovered that lower levels of serotonin
underlie the mild loss of cognitive functions that usually
precede the onset of Alzheimer's.
These findings suggest that preventing the loss of serotonin,
could halt or even prevent,
the progression of Alzheimer's disease and potentially other dementias.

I agree 100%.
Please keep reading so as to learn how to reduce these risks—and so much more.

PART 1

The
Serotonin-Insulin Connection
Revealed

LEARN HOW TO IMPLEMENT THIS SCIENCE

SO YOU CAN

PREVENT AND/OR REVERSE

THE MOST COMMON DISEASES

So,

are you tired of being overweight?

Are you fed up with failing at every diet you've tried?

Are you sick of being called lazy and weak-willed?

Are you done crying yourself to sleep at night?

Are you through being ashamed to go out in public?

Wouldn't you like to know what causes cravings?

Better yet, wouldn't you like to learn how to control your cravings?

Wouldn't you like to know why certain food gives you such emotional comfort?

Wouldn't you like to know why your willpower is never enough?

Wouldn't you like to know why, no matter how much fat free food you eat,
the pounds keep creeping on?

Wouldn't you like to know why, no matter how hard you workout,
you still don't have the body you desire?

Wouldn't you like to know why you're so often moody,
depressed, angry, anxious, and unable to sleep?

Wouldn't you like to know why you have to start your day
with caffeine—and end it with wine?

Wouldn't you like to know why, no matter how healthy you think you're eating,
you have high blood pressure, you're borderline diabetic, with abnormal blood panels?

Wouldn't you like to know why nearly every child suddenly has ADD/ADHD?

Wouldn't you like to know why "high cholesterol" is considered
to be one of the greatest medical scams?

Wouldn't you like to reduce your risks for dementia and Alzheimer's?

Are you fed up with the lies?

More importantly, are you ready for the truth?

Are you willing to make a change, to put forth the required effort?

Are you ready to make the commitment?

Are you ready to make yourself, and your health, a priority?

I sincerely hope so, because this is the answer you've been waiting for.

Be prepared.

Your life is about to be forever changed.

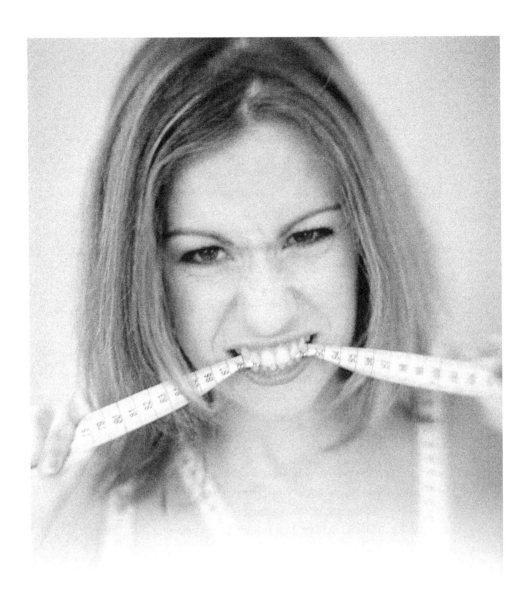

1

WHY 98% OF ALL DIETS FAIL
The missing link needed to overcome obesity

You've certainly caught my attention, but let's get right to the point, shall we? What is this "missing link" you speak of?
It is a fact, and an alarming reality, that 98% of all attempts to lose weight, be it, low cal, low fat, or low carb diets, even stomach stapling—inevitably fail. However, the truth is, these diet failures are not due to lack of willpower, food addiction, or emotional attach-ment. The truth is, diet failure is not your fault. That's right. It's not your fault. Do you really think anyone chooses to be overweight? Obese? Do you really think anyone would intentionally keep failing at every single diet? Of course not. Diet failure, in most cases, is not your fault.

Yeah, right! It's not my fault? Please! Are you kidding or what?
First of all, please understand that the mere word "diet" implies someone is, in fact, at least trying. And no, I'm not kidding. I'm very serious. To be able to tell someone that diet failure is not their fault is so empowering. Whereas everyone else would love for you to believe it's about willpower, mind control, determination, starvation, deprivation, or food addictions, I'm going to tell you something that will change your life forever—and free you from the tortured guilt of having failed at so many diets in the past.

Haven't you ever wondered *why* it's so hard to stick to a healthy way of eating? Haven't you ever wondered *why,* no matter how many times, in how many ways, health experts tell you what to eat to lose the weight, you simply cannot stick to their diets? Haven't you ever wondered *why* cravings are always your downfall? Haven't you ever wondered *why* all your diets have failed?

Of course you have. We all have. Time after time, you start a diet with all the passion, conviction, and promises that you'll succeed. You vow to do whatever it takes, and as long as it takes, to lose the weight. Considering you're far from being a quitter, you begin each new diet with this same intensity. You're off to a great start. Eating low-calorie, then low-fat, now it's low carb. You're not really sure what to eat anymore, but you are com-mitted like never before.

Sadly, only weeks, maybe months into it, you find yourself sabotaging this diet as well. Chip by chip. Cookie by cookie. You find it impossible to resist the carbs that have always given you such comfort. With each loss of control, the pounds start to creep back on.

Whatever weight you lost, you've gained back—and more! *But why?* Why is it so hard? It's not like you're incompetent. After all, you're successful in your career. You have a happy and fulfilling marriage with three beautiful children, so why is it you can't succeed at losing some lousy weight and keep it off?

Wouldn't you like to know why all your best intentions have never been enough? Wouldn't you like to know why food has always controlled you? Wouldn't you like to know why, no matter how hard you train, you still don't have the body that you really desire? Aren't you tired of people assuming you're overweight because you're weak-willed, lazy, or unwilling? *Don't you want to know why all your diets have failed?*

Yes! Of course I do!
First of all, diets fail for two simple, yet crucial, reasons: cravings and appetite. Most of us hopefully realize by now that our shocking rate of obesity is not due to eating healthy fat, but due, rather, to eating the wrong type of and/or far too many carbohydrates. And though we can be told all day long what NOT to eat to stay lean and healthy, it is entirely another matter to *control* the insatiable carb/sugar cravings and overall appetite. Hence, the astounding 98% rate of diet failure.

You're exactly right. I have no willpower! I feel like I'm addicted to certain carbs. But why can't I control my cravings?
Unlike what so many others have told you through the years, it's not your fault that you can't stick to those diets. In most cases, it's not your fault that you're overweight. While you'll most certainly have to at least make an effort to eat healthy, successful dieting has absolutely nothing to do with a lack of willpower, nor is it about food intolerances, having to starve yourself, or using stimulants. And, it is most assuredly <u>not</u> about being addicted to certain carbs, though, that is precisely how it feels.

Can't I just not worry about my lack of willpower and get my stomach stapled like so many others are doing?
I suppose you can do anything you want. But unless your weight has gotten to the point where it means life or death, I would seriously recommend you reconsider. Gastric bypass surgery is an extremely risky procedure and should be considered only if you need to lose 200 pounds or more. And, while its goal is to severely reduce the amount of food the patient can take in, you need to realize that it is only a temporary fix. It's only masking the underlying problem.

So, what is your solution? What is the missing link? Please tell me!
Are you sure you want to know? Are you really ready to take this information and utilize it? With all due respect, even though I've now shared this research with thousands of people, there's a certain percentage who choose to totally disregard it, who are unwilling to make the necessary changes in lifestyle, and who, instead, keep silently praying for that ever-elusive magic diet pill. I'm sorry, but if you don't know it already, that magic pill does <u>not</u>

exist. Therefore, your success will require effort. So, again I ask: Are you ready to take this information and actually *utilize* it? Sadly, even some of my clients refuse to do so.

Yes, I'm very serious. I'm ready! Please, I want to know!
The truth is that successful, i.e., *long-term* weight loss is, in fact, based on "BRAIN CHEMISTRY." The answer, the solution, the missing (and crucial) link that most experts have missed, is that 98% of all diets fail due to the depletion of a very precise brain chemical.

Excuse me? A brain chemical?
Yes, a brain chemical. That extraordinary, extremely powerful major neurotransmitter is called serotonin (5-hydroxytryptamine, 5-HT). Stronger than any street drug, serotonin is the most important neurotransmitter, the master communicator among the many other brain chemicals. The serotonin system is the largest single system in the brain. It's also abundant in the digestive system. Therefore, for your mind and body to work at its very best, *to function as effectively as possible*, serotonin levels must be maintained. Serotonin, though, is also the brain chemical that has clinically proven to control the two major reasons why diets inevitably fail. To finally understand that successful weight loss is based on brain chemistry, not willpower or addiction, is the most empowering information that I can share with my clients. Without a doubt, it's the research everyone needs to learn about. It will empower people as never before. It will free them of the endless and senseless shame over all their failed diets.

Are you serious? My inability to stick with a diet is not about being weak-willed?
This is exactly what I'm saying. Successful weight loss is based on maintaining healthy levels of serotonin. And healthy levels of serotonin will, subsequently, lead to controlling insulin levels. This **"Serotonin-Insulin Connection"** is the crucial link for achieving successful weight loss. (I explain this in much greater detail in the following chapters.)

All this time, I've felt like such a loser! I'm ashamed at how many diets I've failed at. But why isn't anyone else talking about this?
Most people only know of serotonin and its relation to depression. They have no clue as to its extraordinary abilities to control carb/sugar cravings and overall appetite. Nor do I hear anyone in the media discussing the direct correlation to low serotonin and anxiety, bulimia, insomnia, ADD/ADHD, OCD, rage, alcoholism, migraines, transfer of addictions, Alzheimer's, etc. All these reasons, and many more, are why it's so important for me to get this information to the masses. It gives people the answer, the *solution* they've been searching for. It explains in precise, yet simple detail, exactly *why* all their past diets have failed. It also explains why they may be moody, depressed, anxious, angry, unable to concentrate or sleep, etc. While the information I am about to share with you is based on sound clinical science, it's extremely easy to comprehend. When I share this research with my clients, the light suddenly goes on. They finally get it.

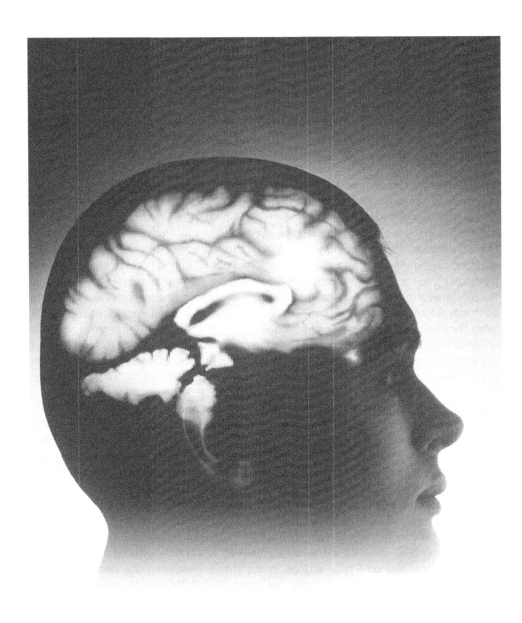

2

SEROTONIN:
AN EXTRAORDINARY BRAIN CHEMICAL
A carb addict you are not

Can you please tell me again what serotonin is?
Serotonin is the most important neurotransmitter, a brain chemical, that regulates food cravings, satiety (appetite), mood, sleep, pain, aggression, anxiety, and much more.

What causes cravings?
Cravings are due to low serotonin levels. When this brain chemical gets depleted, we *subconsciously* crave the types of food that breakdown quickly into blood sugar, i.e., high glycemic index (GI) carbohydrates. These particular carbs range from bagels, white bread, pasta, pastries, chips, crackers, candy, cereal, sodas, fruit juices, etc. These carbs spike insulin levels. Insulin, allows tryptophan to cross the blood brain barrier. Tryptophan transforms into serotonin. And serotonin. . . *makes us feel good!* These carbs have, subsequently, become known as "comfort food." This is why people tend to eat out of emotion. This chemical shift in the brain, though subtle, makes us feel good. Simply put, people eat these particular carbs to feel better. They are, in fact, self-medicating. So you see, there is indeed an emotional attachment and reward to this eating pattern. Unfortunately, this is exactly why our obesity rate is as high as it is.

That's ironic. Isn't this how low fat food makes you feel?
Yes. While fat free/low fat food may be low in fat, they are, instead, loaded with sugar, causing the same response. Furthermore, though carbs like bagels, bread, cereal, and pasta are usually fat free/low fat and generally considered complex carbs, they're highly refined so as to give them that oooh, so delicious taste; especially bagels to make them ever so moist. It's this process that makes them high GI carbs. *Why?* Because refined/processed carbs need relatively no digestion time. Therefore, the minute you eat them, they immediately breakdown into blood sugar. This causes your insulin levels to rise rapidly. You're actually better off eating food that still contains healthy fat. Also, this fat free/high carb food contains little, if any, real nutritional value.

Once again, when serotonin is depleted, cravings sneak in. Eating these high GI and/or excessive carbohydrates causes a rapid release of insulin. While one of insulin's roles is to carefully regulate the amount of blood sugar going to the brain, the increased levels of insulin will also boost serotonin levels. And it's serotonin that makes us feel so damn good. But, this feeling of comfort we get from these carbs is merely temporary, lasting an hour or so. To get that feeling again, our brain forces us, on a subconscious level, to eat more of the same. Once again, insulin spiking leads to the production of serotonin. This cycle is repeated over and over. Day after day. Month after month. While the effects of serotonin are short-lived, the excess insulin, which will make your body store fat each and every time it's spiked, is not. The result: a nation that is 45% obese and depressed. Since COVID, and now the far deadlier strain, Delta, those numbers will go much higher. FACT: 98% of all diets will inevitably fail, unless you're able to maintain healthy levels of serotonin.

I swear I'm addicted to bread! And I sure do love my chips!
Unfortunately, there are far too many people who believe it's about being addicted to this type of food. This is not true. It is, though, about this vital brain chemical being depleted. The only addiction is, wanting to self-medicate by eating the high GI carbs that trigger the increase of serotonin, all of which is done on a subconscious level.

With no desire to ever speak out of turn, we've all heard Oprah speak about her carb addiction. She once said, "I'm no different than any other type of addict." She said this was simply who she was and she'd have to accept it. I wanted to cry in frustration, because her addiction to carbs is merely due to *low serotonin*. I was desperate to share my research with her, to help her understand why she craves certain carbs and how to control her carb addiction once and for all.

There are millions who feel like her. I'm addicted to chocolate!
I know, but it's NOT YOUR FAULT. It's about understanding what happens when serotonin is depleted. It's also about a level of commitment. If I may be so bold, far too many people bitch and moan endlessly about being overweight. Unfortunately, they aren't willing to make the commitment that's required to achieve a leaner, healthier body. Oprah is committed to training. However, her journey could've been far easier had she been aware of this science. Maybe one day I will be fortunate enough to share my expertise with her. I would mitigate her carb addiction in mere days. No more guilt. No more failed diets.

UPDATE, A FATHER'S LOVE: My father was so impressed with my work. He wrote Oprah a letter, telling her I was doing more for my clients than any doctor could. To our surprise, in less than 14 days, one of her producers called. She was impressed with my book and requested a copy. We were so excited! However, one year to the day that letter was penned, Oprah announced she was back up to 200 pounds. She admitted she continues to struggle with her carb addictions. She spoke of her embarrassment over allowing this to happen again. Her staff had my book for 10 long months, a book that would explain, and put an end to, Oprah's cravings, plus, so much more. I was beyond frustrated.

I can certainly relate to anyone who struggles with cravings, after all, my cravings used to be for sourdough bread, diet sodas, and alcohol. And, no amount of willpower could stop me from consuming those things, once my serotonin dropped. Back in the day, when I didn't know much about nutrition, and absolutely nothing about serotonin, my serotonin was always low. But once I went into R&D and studied serotonin, and all the side effects of low serotonin, moreover, how to safely elevate and maintain this vital brain chemical, my life completely changed.

Fascinating! Isn't bread a starchy carb, a carb that you want us to avoid? Either way, I need help controlling my cravings, too.
Yes, it's a starchy carb and a very common comfort food. Read on. You'll gain the knowledge needed to live a much healthier lifestyle. You'll learn how to maintain your serotonin levels, thereby, controlling the ever-powerful carb cravings. You'll also learn why all this low fat/fat free food has made you heavier than ever, depressed, addicted, etc.

A low fat/fat free diet = high carb/sugar = high insulin = excess body fat.

What else does serotonin control?
Serotonin is a major neurotransmitter that not only controls carbohydrate cravings, but also naturally reduces appetite, as it's the satiety control mechanism for the body.

Serotonin controls my appetite, as well as my cravings?
Yes. It's one thing to control cravings, but your total caloric intake also plays an essential role in lifelong weight loss. The most basic concept of weight loss is: Eating more calories than your body requires will be stored as fat. This is predominantly true with an excess of carbohydrates, because carbs cannot be used for anything except to fuel the body. Thus, if they're not used, they will be promoted to fat storage. Whereas with protein and fat, the body can utilize the excess for rebuilding the body's cells, hormones, enzymes, muscles, neurotransmitters, etc. Once again, serotonin naturally controls the two key reasons why diets fail: Carbohydrate cravings and appetite.

Healthy levels of serotonin are also crucial to alleviating depression, anxiety, panic attacks, stress, headaches, migraines, pain, PMS, ADD, OCD, etc. Once you're able to achieve and maintain healthy serotonin levels, you will not only start to lose the excess weight, but your mood will also be fantastic. You'll feel less stressed. Sleep patterns will improve greatly. You'll be slower to anger, calmer, and more focused. Body aches and pain will be reduced. You'll have far more energy, without having to use harmful stimulants. Your entire life will be more focused and energized. Serotonin controls so many amazing functions within the body. I insist, though, that my clients do not take my word for it, but, instead, research it on their own. Then, they will truly understand serotonin's extensive health benefits.

How does serotonin become depleted?
Basically everything in life seems to deplete serotonin, ranging from stress, lack of deep restorative (quality) sleep, poor nutrition, sedentary lifestyle, low fat dieting and dieting in general, high GI and excessive carbohydrate consumption, processed/refined food, sugar, and artificial sweeteners. Caffeine, nicotine, ephedra, chocolate, alcohol, over-the-counter meds, and prescription and nonprescription drugs all deplete serotonin, as well.

Oh, my! All of those things deplete serotonin?
Yes, and it's a vicious cycle. *Why?* Because who doesn't have stress in their life? How often do you eat balanced, nutritious meals? When's the last time you had a quality night's sleep? And who doesn't drink coffee or alcohol? All these things, plus numerous others, deplete serotonin. We then become depressed. Irritable. Anxious. Stressed. Quick to anger. Tired. We look for emotional relief. Anything to make us feel better. Our minds then *subconsciously* force us toward the types of food and/or substances that it knows will stimulate the production of serotonin, thereby, making us feel good. Most of us don't even know why we crave chocolate cake, mac' and cheese, potato chips, bagels, or even caffeine and alcohol. We just assume we're weak, addicted, or without willpower. Not true. Cravings are a side of effect of low serotonin. Critical fact: Elevating serotonin in this manner, requires a spike in insulin. And insulin is the hormone that causes the body to store fat.

Is this why I find myself craving carbs after a long, stressful day?
Exactly. In addition to the high stress level, you've probably also consumed many of the other things that equally deplete serotonin. By day's end, your serotonin has plummeted. Your brain then begins to create noise, i.e., cravings. And it will continually force you to seek the carbs that it knows will, once again, trigger the production of this crucial, ever-comforting brain chemical. For those who have ever had a craving, including myself, you know only too well just how powerful they can be. They are not to be ignored. To reiterate, brain chemicals are stronger than any street drug, and when the brain thinks it's starving, it will do anything and everything to save itself. Hence, it forces you to consume the carbs that breakdown quickest into blood sugar. Its other critical goal is to boost serotonin, no matter how brief, so as to help the body/mind function properly.

Cravings are merely a side effect of low serotonin.

Another example is when you don't get enough sleep. Haven't you ever noticed when you're tired, maybe after a night out or merely a restless night's sleep, and the only food you seem to be hungry for are carbs? No matter how hard you try to avoid them, *nothing* satisfies your appetite. That is, not until you finally take a bite of your favorite carb. Maybe it's pizza. Cereal. Sweet potato pie. Pasta. Toasted bagel. Pretzels. French fries. Or maybe you lean more toward ice cream. Dried fruit. Yogurt. Raisins. Wine. Oreo cookies. Chocolate bar. Nonetheless, whatever your carb selection, once consumed, *once you've spiked your insulin*, the increase in serotonin is soon to follow. Ooooh, that feeling of comfort is only moments away! Like magic, the cravings suddenly stop. Your hunger ceases. You sit back, take a deep breath, you feel soooo good! Well, at least for an hour or so. But there they are. Once again. The cravings come gently knocking. Then screaming. Until you give in. The cycle repeats. Over and over.

This is so true! I can't believe it! This is exactly what happens to me when I don't get enough sleep. It's only after I eat one of my favorite carbs that I feel content.
The comfort you derive from eating high GI carbs is definitely short-lived. Once your sero-

tonin drops again, which it will within about an hour, your brain will start the craving cycle all over again. Don't forget, each time that you give in to these cravings, you're causing your body to store more fat. So, yes, insomnia is another side effect of low serotonin. But please don't take Ambien, Lunesta or any other drug to induce sleep. Not only are these drugs addictive, but the side effects are insane, ranging from preparing/consuming meals, having sex, even driving a car, and all without any memory. Instead of taking drugs, make sure you have enough serotonin throughout the day to *convert* to melatonin come the sleep cycle. (Still can't sleep? Try taking 200mg of 5-HTP at bedtime.)

I could definitely use better sleep. So, where is serotonin found?
Serotonin is produced in different parts of the brain and body where it can be stored or released. Although most of the body's serotonin is found in the gastrointestinal system and in blood platelets, its most well-known effects are in the brain. The activity of serotonin arises in the brainstem from clusters of neurons known as the raphe nucleus. From the brain, serotonin neurons extend to virtually all parts of the CNS (Central Nervous System) making the branching of the serotonin network the most expansive neurochemical system in the brain. The importance of this network becomes quite apparent when you realize that each and every serotonin neuron exerts an influence over as many as 500,000 target neurons. Due to this vast distribution of serotonin in the CNS, it's not surprising that this neurotransmitter is linked to so many types of behavior.

Wow! Amazing information! So where does serotonin actually come from?
The most important raw ingredient is an amino acid called tryptophan. Tryptophan is naturally found in dietary protein. It's essential for the production of serotonin. When you eat a fat free/low fat diet, the often feared, but purported fatty food such as red meat, eggs, nuts, avocados, poultry, and cheese (which are also healthy sources of protein), are often eliminated from your diet. By doing this, you have robbed your body of the raw materials needed to produce adequate amounts of tryptophan. Without enough tryptophan, your body can't naturally produce enough serotonin.

What are the side effects of serotonin deficiency?
There are numerous side effects when serotonin is deficient. However, the side effects that contribute to diet failure are cravings and binge eating, particularly for the kind of carbs that breakdown quickly into blood sugar. And, as you've just learned, those carbs are known as simple/high GI carbs. Depression and anxiety are also common side effects.

Depression, as well? Any other side effects?
Depression is due to serotonin being depleted (no matter the underlying cause), especially when it's low on a constant basis. (Magnesium deficiency can also cause depression and anxiety.) As for other side effects, most people I share this information with are shocked to realize just how many health conditions are directly related to low serotonin. (Or as the FDA and drug companies would like to call them: diseases.) Nevertheless, people need to understand that serotonin is a "MAJOR NEUROTRANSMITTER" and, as such, when

it's out of balance, your entire body and mind will suffer in various ways. So, yes, in addition to carb/sugar cravings, binge eating, insomnia, and depression, other side effects would include obesity, rage, sudden outbursts, mood swings, ADD/ADHD, extreme agitation, anxiety, panic attacks, PMS, alcoholism, headaches, migraines, repetitive behavior, chronic body pain, low energy, lack of creative focus, decreased sex drive (yes, *decreased* sex drive), irritable bowel syndrome, memory loss, transfer of addictions, schizophrenia, and suicidal behavior. Recent studies suggest that serotonin also plays a role in endocrine regulation, muscle contraction, cardiovascular function, stroke, hypertension, and our ability to learn.

I would never have believed that serotonin could control so many things.
Yes, serotonin undeniably controls all these things, and many more. Therefore, when this brain chemical is depleted, countless health conditions will arise. Side effects will vary from person to person. They also vary in degree depending upon whether or not serotonin levels are fluctuated quickly versus if they're constantly low.

So how do I achieve and maintain healthy levels of serotonin naturally?
For starters, you need to provide your body with balanced nutrition, regular exercise, and quality sleep. These things will help provide healthy serotonin levels. A diet that contains plenty of food rich in tryptophan, i.e., fresh fish, meat, milk, eggs, turkey, and nuts, may also be helpful in boosting serotonin. Unfortunately, it would be extremely difficult to eat enough of this food to supply the needed tryptophan. In addition, you must also eliminate all stress, stimulants, recreational drugs, high GI and excessive carbohydrate consumption, sugar, artificial sweeteners, prescription and nonprescription drugs, nicotine, caffeine, alcohol, and any other insulin-releasing factors. Add to that the fact that most people live sedentary lives, and it's easy to understand why it's nearly impossible to maintain healthy serotonin levels on our own. Based on the lifestyle of most Americans, we are a nation that is, without a doubt, suffering from what is now being recognized as "Serotonin Deficiency Syndrome."

What are the benefits of healthy serotonin levels?
The health benefits are truly endless. To begin with, when the brain has healthy levels of serotonin, it will stop demanding outside substances, i.e., high GI carbohydrates, sugar, caffeine, nicotine, alcohol, etc., that stimulate a quick release of serotonin. Properly balanced serotonin levels will also provide a tremendous sense of well-being, contentment, and happiness. It will energize your life, promote deep restorative sleep, diminish anxiety and stress, alleviate pain, ADD/ADHD, PMS, as well as enhance your sense of focus, mental clarity, creativity, productivity, and sexual behavior. As you can see, serotonin is absolutely crucial to your mental and physical health.

It seems low serotonin levels are displayed in different ways?
This is precisely what happens. Through the years, our brains have become conditioned to know exactly what will elevate our serotonin. Some people will crave corn bread, chips,

biscuits, or cereal. Others may crave chocolate, juice, or sodas. Some will crave alcohol or caffeine. Still others may crave cigarettes. *Each person exhibits low serotonin levels in their own unique way.* To reiterate, we each have unknowingly conditioned our brain through our lifetime of eating habits. However, to crave anything is a sign of low serotonin. It's also a sign of being unhealthy. And, to those who say they "don't have cravings," it doesn't necessarily have to be an overwhelming urge. It's simply the types of food you are *drawn* to, and they'll most often be high GI carbs, i.e., food that triggers insulin.

Is this why I feel so depressed when I diet?
Most often, yes. Fat free/low fat dieting is the biggest contributor to this, as it eliminates the precise food that the body needs to make adequate amounts of serotonin.

How will low carb dieting affect my mood?
People will unquestionably feel their moods spiral downward, as they will no longer be consuming the high GI carbs that so easily triggered the production of serotonin. They'll also feel more stressed, anxious, unable to concentrate, etc. And this is when the cravings kick in. Because the brain is perfectly conditioned to know what it needs, it will literally force you toward the carbs/beverages that it knows will elevate this powerful brain chemical. Your brain will create this noise until you give in. It will force you to eat the types of carbs, i.e., bread, chips, candy, sodas, fast food, etc., that will once again elevate serotonin. The result: you'll feel great! Unfortunately, it will also make you FAT. Now, more than ever, people need to realize that unless they're able to maintain adequate serotonin levels, all attempts at dieting will fail, especially low carb dieting. This is exactly why most diets fail. It's one thing to tell people what not to eat; it's another matter entirely for them to adhere to that diet regimen if their serotonin is low. This is particularly important when it concerns controlling cravings and/or desires for sugar/carbs, because it's these precise carbs that cause the body to store fat.

My eating habits are fine in the morning. In fact, I rarely eat breakfast.
Most people, especially women, feel that the less they eat, the thinner they will be. Not true. This is a far too common misconception. This is a classic example of low calorie dieting—and low calorie dieting will only set you up for more weight gain. Then, there are others who complain that by eating breakfast, they're much hungrier throughout the day so they, too, skip breakfast, eat a late lunch on the run, and then, come dinner time, when they're basically starving, they inhale whatever is put before them. More often than not, either scenario will lead to people consuming far too much food for that late hour. Regardless, that one large meal at the end of the day is not generally enough to make people gain fat. Those who attempt to lose weight this way must wonder *why* they're gaining weight. After all, they only ate one meal, and even though the meal was late in the day, it was far from an "excess" of calories. So, why can't they lose weight? Moreover, why are they gaining weight so fast? Allow me to explain:

1) When you don't properly fuel your body throughout the day, your serotonin will plum-

met. Low serotonin will cause cravings for high GI carbs and binge eating. Hence, your only desire at the end of your long stressed out day will be to eat processed/refined/starchy carbs and lots of them, because the body is desperate to raise this crucial brain chemical. And the quickest way to achieve this is by eating high GI carbs. Unfortunately, these particular carbs will spike insulin, forcing them directly into fat storage. Even if you were to workout with hopes to burn off the excessive sugar caused by these high GI carbs, it's never healthy to spike your insulin. Plus, you can NEVER out-train your diet.

2) If your serotonin is low, which is most certain, you'll be more likely to eat the wrong types of food late day. So, maintain your serotonin with the 5. This will control your cravings and appetite. Then, I highly recommend Intermittent Fasting, which is all about a controlled set of time that you eat. The health benefits from fasting are remarkable!

No wonder I can't lose weight. I'll start eating breakfast and I'll try fasting. But I'm still confused. Why do my cravings for chocolate only come late in the day?
Depending on your quality of sleep, your cravings generally should be nonexistent upon rising. This is because your body is able to replenish some of your serotonin as you sleep. As a result, when you get up, you should feel rested, ready to go, minus any cravings. As the day goes on, though, you will endure endless degrees of stress. While stress alone can play complete havoc on serotonin, you'll be exposed to many other contributing factors. They can range from cereal, skim milk, fruit juice, donuts, bagels, mocha frappuccino, latte drizzled with a sugary syrup, toast, sodas, chips, pizza, fries, a midday candy bar with a cigarette, and another latte. All in the same day, you find out your teenager has been skipping school, your boss is on a rampage, your car needs work, and your husband is going out of town, again. As you prepare to tackle the long commute home, you drink some orange juice, taking three extra strength Excedrin with the hope that they will help alleviate your throbbing headache. Ahhh, another day!

Whew! That sounds just like my life!
I know. Unfortunately, this is a very common description of how most Americans get through their day. It is also a mere example of some of the many things that we ingest, and endure, from day to day. Nonetheless, each and every one of those things depletes serotonin. This is why, by day's end, your serotonin is bottomed out. It's amazing chocolate is all you reach for. And, you go for sweets, because your brain is long conditioned to know that chocolate is *your* drug of choice, so to speak. Your brain knows that chocolate is what will boost your serotonin. I'm sure you started this behavior many years ago, probably as a young girl. Consequently, your brain starts to create this craving, and it will continually force you toward chocolate, because it knows, from years of experience, that this is what elevates your serotonin. Your comfort food just happens to be chocolate.

You're right, chocolate has always been my comfort food. Now I finally know *why* I can't live without it. I guess serotonin really is the key to successful fat loss!
Without a doubt, you need to maintain healthy levels of all your brain chemicals for opti-

mum health, but serotonin, the master communicator of all brain chemicals, is the crucial link to successful weight loss, as it controls the cravings for the type of carbs that trigger insulin and cause the body to store fat, while at the same time controlling overall appetite.

Chocolate is *your* drug of choice.

This is fascinating, but I love my chocolate. What if I'm not ready to give it up?
Ah, L-O-V-E! Or so you think. This is an excellent comment, as I have counseled many a client who has said the exact same thing. While you may think you "love and need" your chocolate (wine, beer, pasta, bread, etc.), what you're actually so in love with is the feeling of *comfort* you get after eating it. It is the emotional relief that always follows after you eat chocolate that has you so attached to this sweet, creamy delight. It is this act of self-medicating that gets you into this addictive behavior pattern. It is the elevation in the wonderful, mood-altering brain chemical serotonin that makes you hesitant, if not fearful, to give it up. You need to understand, though, there is a huge difference between simply wanting something versus *having* to have it at all cost. Those costs are your health and well-being. I'm not saying you can never eat chocolate again. I'm trying to make you understand why you feel so attached to it. It's the same for someone who is attached to pasta, pastries, chips, dumplings, soda, alcohol, caffeine, and nicotine.

How will I know the difference?
Easy. One of the most rewarding aspects of maintaining healthy levels of serotonin is that you will no longer be controlled by these cravings. You will be able to get through the day and night <u>without</u> needing (*or even thinking about*) these insulin-producing carbs. Your once insatiable desire or "love" for chocolate will simply vanish. You'll be amazed at how easily this happens. I guarantee you.

Are you sure I won't miss my chocolate? I've never been able to give it up.
The only reason your mind continuously tempts you with chocolate is, because your serotonin is, unquestionably, deficient. But once you maintain healthy levels of serotonin, your craving for this comfort food will disappear. *Why?* Because your brain will become satiated. Hence, the noise, i.e., craving, will stop. Your brain will no longer need to force you toward this high GI carb that has faithfully boosted your serotonin for years. Unlike every other diet you've ever tried before, your cravings and appetite will be controlled *without* any sense of frustration, deprivation, or starvation. You will be in complete control. Without effort. Without the usual emotional drama and struggle. You will come to fully understand that this desperate, so-called love affair with chocolate is NOT about love, after all. It is, though, merely a "side effect" of low serotonin. It is at this time that you will finally be free of this food addiction. It is, once again, the **"Serotonin-Insulin Connection"** that is absolutely vital to achieving and maintaining, among many things, your weight loss goals.

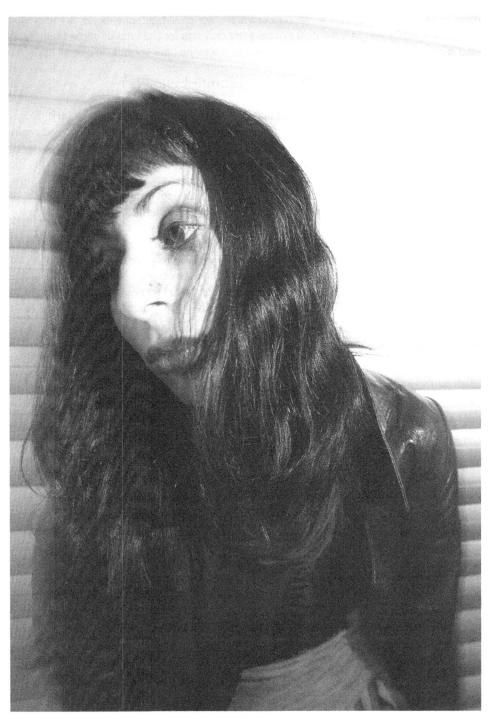

3

OH, THE MANY DIETS WE'VE FALLEN PREY TO
From starvation to the low fat myth

All this time I thought eating low calorie or low fat were the answer.
Contrary to these theories that the AMA (American Medical Association), AHA (American Heart Association), and FDA (Food and Drug Administration) preached to us for 40+ years, they just did not work. In fact, as a nation, we got fatter than ever before. This diet regime has caused an epidemic of alarming obesity-related health conditions.

Why don't these diets work?
<u>Low calorie dieting:</u>
Your body interprets a low calorie diet as starvation. This includes skipping meals and eating bare minimum. (Meal replacement bars/drinks fall under the bare minimum category and they're perfect examples of severe caloric restriction. And don't let anyone put you on Medifast.) You'll lose weight at first, as your glycogen stores are depleted, but your weight loss will plateau. Then the real damage begins. Your body instinctively reacts with a survival mechanism that is intended to prevent loss of lean muscle and bone mass. Instead of burning fat, your body will actually start to *hoard* fat. The less you eat, the slower your metabolism, the slower your bodily functions become. Your body will eventually start consuming its own tissue in order to get the nutrients that it needs to sustain the most vital body part: *your brain*. This type of dieting actually changes the overall composition of your body. With each diet, you'll <u>lose</u> more lean muscle and bone mass, while at the same time *increasing* fat storage. The less lean muscle tissue, the less efficient your body is at burning fat. Thus, the all too common diet scenario: "Lose 10/gain back 20."

So skipping meals is not good?
If you're eating healthy, with plenty of fat and protein, water, etc., then missing a meal or two can be very beneficial, as with intermittent fasting. (Personally, I love fasting 18-22 hours every day.) But when you don't properly fuel your brain, *which will do whatever it takes to stay alive*, it will struggle—and cravings are just the beginning.

<u>Fat free/low fat dieting:</u>
I call this the low fat *myth*, as there was not one long-term study that verified the efficacy of such a diet. If this diet really worked, why, then, is everyone fatter (and sicker) than ever?

FACT: Eating healthy dietary fat does NOT cause the body to store fat, because it does NOT trigger the insulin response. Plus, if you're eating a low fat diet, you're definitely eating too many carbs, which equals too much sugar. It's by eating high GI carbs, processed/refined carbs, and/or an excess of carbs, that is the underlying cause of obesity.

Are you saying butter won't make me fat?
Precisely, which is why people are so confused as to what to eat. Once again, eating healthy fat does not make you fat, because it does not trigger the release of insulin, the fat storing/fat building hormone. Eat an abundance of heathy fat every day.

FAT FACTS: It's necessary for optimum health and reproduction. It supplies essential fatty acids for growth, healthy skin, vitamin absorption, and regulation of bodily functions. Building blocks of cells. Provides more energy than carbs, and slows down the transient time of food, thus lowering GI of carbs. The body needs fat to burn fat. Low fat diets produce high levels of insulin, accelerate metabolic aging process, slow down metabolism, cause weight gain, high BP, thyroid issues, heart attacks, and insulin resistance, which will lead to type 2 diabetes, etc. Summary? A low fat diet will make you fat—and sick.

Eating healthy fat does NOT make you fat.

Still not convinced? Okay, forget about the lack of studies and/or the basic physiology of how the body works. Here's some hard evidence: 100% of the people I consult with are 20 to 200+ pounds overweight. 100% of those clients are all eating based on the low fat myth. (UPDATE: A client shared my research with his doctor. The physician was very impressed, but admitted he had "no idea that insulin had anything to do with fat storage." He then looked it up. He was surprised to see that I was correct. Amazing.)

Amazing, is right! If not, disturbing. What's considered a healthy fat?
Healthy fats are found in nature. They can include meat, butter, heavy whipping cream, eggs, olives, avocado oil mayo, cheese, poultry, fish, oils, nuts, seeds, and avocados. You should eat healthy fats with every meal. Extra virgin olive, walnut, coconut, and macadamia nut oils are recommended. (Best fats to cook with are butter, ghee, coconut, macadamia nut, and avocado oils.) Good fats are known as the essential fatty acids (EFAs), which include omega-3s, omega-6s, and omega-9s, each are crucial to maintaining good health, more so, omega-3s. Mackerel, salmon, anchovies, sardines, herring, tuna, caviar, cod liver and cod liver oil are all rich in omega-3s. Eggs, sunflower and safflower oils, turkey, and chicken are all healthy sources of omega-6s. Omega-9s include oleic acid, which can come from olive and avocado oils, walnuts and almonds. Fats to avoid: man-made fats such as hydrogenated/trans fats and oils which are found in fries, chips, cookies, pastries, certain meats, margarine products, and even some alleged health products.

I hear all this talk about avoiding "trans fats," but I'm not sure what they are?
Trans fats are basically fats that are "transformed" from their natural state. They are unsaturated fatty acids formed when vegetable oils are processed and made more solid. This processing is called hydrogenation. Avoid trans fats.

WARNING: Fat Free/Low Fat Food Alert: Fat free/low fat food are loaded with sugar. When you take the fat out of food, you take out the flavor. To enhance the flavor, food companies add sugar. They add a lot, and they add the worst kind: high-fructose corn syrup. (They also add chemicals and salt. Salt causes water retention, which equals more weight gain.) High-fructose corn syrup is more harmful than table sugar. It accelerates the metabolic aging process more than any form of sugar. It depletes serotonin. Encourages the body to store fat. Perpetuates carbohydrate cravings. It's addictive. A vicious and unhealthy cycle of cravings, excessive fat gain, and low serotonin levels are fueled by fat free/low fat diets.

What about fat free yogurt? Aren't they okay?
No. All you have to do is read the nutrition label to see just how much sugar is in one of those tiny containers. Dannon: A 6 oz. container has 33g of carbs; a staggering 30g of those carbs are SUGAR. Yoplait Whips shamefully contains fructose, high-fructose corn syrup, corn starch, and dextrose, totaling 23g of sugar in a mere 4 oz. Yoplait Light contains aspartame—and proudly lists it right on the front panel. And, because most yogurts are "fat free," they'll affect blood sugar levels that much quicker. Without any fat, and all that fruit sugar, it's going to spike your insulin, putting your body into a fat-storing mode.

With regard to drinkable yogurts, they're even worse, due to the mere fact they're a *liquid* carb. Liquid carbs affect your blood sugar levels so much faster than solid carbs. They also have just as many carbs/sugars, if not more, than the original yogurts. Example: Dannon's Fruision, 10 oz., has 52g of carbs; 49g of those carbs are sugar. Yoplait Nouriche, another liquid yogurt, at 11 ounces, has an astounding 60g of carbs; 46g of those carbs are sugar. It also contains high-fructose corn syrup. This product is one of the worst. And with absolutely zero fat, it's nothing more than liquid sugar. Yoplait's marketing campaign would like us to believe that this is the perfect healthy breakfast food for those on the run. Wrong. This is not a healthy choice for a meal, let alone the first thing you put into your body.

Fruit contains fructose, i.e., FRUIT SUGAR.

And smoothies, aren't they a healthy choice?
Smoothies are a ton of fruit blended, creating a delicious, but nonetheless, purely liquid candy beverage. Drinking a smoothie (or fruit juice), be it with a healthy meal or otherwise, is too much sugar going into the blood stream. This surge of sugar will spike insulin levels, putting the body into a fat-storing mode. It will also deplete serotonin levels, cause mood swings, affect the body's energy levels, etc.

Isn't fruit healthy?
Yes, it is, but it's a simple carb, same family as a candy bar. It contains fructose, fruit sugar, just as milk contains lactose, milk sugar. When you blend fruit, you breakdown the fiber, turning it into pure sugar water. As a liquid carb, it affects blood sugars levels even more dramatically than solid carbs, due to the fact the body doesn't have to break it down.

Liquid carbs are basically sugar, as they go directly into the blood stream, quickly spiking insulin levels. Therefore, the best way to eat fruit is in its natural state. (An apple versus apple juice.) Don't blend it or break it down, and don't eat it first or alone. And whether it's a smoothie, fruit juice, pre-bottled, or you get one from Jamba Juice, they should all come with nutrition information. Read it. You'll see they are extremely high in sugar. Remember, the best way to eat fruit is in its natural state, which keeps the fiber intact, hence, lowering the GI. Also, when trying to shed excess body fat, limit your fruit, low GI or otherwise.

And serotonin is the crucial link to controlling those cravings?

Exactly! I don't want you not to eat carbs, I want you to eat the *right* carbs. This research is about helping people understand why 98% of all diets fail. This research is about helping people understand that their inability to adhere to any such diet is not their fault, but instead due to *cravings* caused by the depletion of a brain chemical. These particular cravings are for the precise carbs that spike insulin levels, causing the body to store fat. By boosting and maintaining your serotonin, the brain chemical that governs carbohydrate cravings and overall appetite, you will finally be able to control the cravings for those insulin-producing carbs. No longer will you be controlled by the food that has always kept you overweight. To sum it up: If you want to reach optimum health, it's not about dieting. It's not about eating low cal or low fat, rather, LOW CARB and HIGHER FAT. It's about fueling your body and brain with the healthiest food possible. It's also about living a healthy lifestyle.

It makes sense, but I'm still confused. What do you eat?

My day starts with a glass of room temp water with fresh lemon and sea salt. Next, a collagen drink to take my take my supps, especially the 5-HTP. Twenty minutes later I typically have 3 eggs, 2 tbsp butter, 1 tbsp EVOO, whole avocado and 1 oz goat cheese, or maybe 3 oz chicken thigh, 2 tbsp EVOO, 1 tbsp ghee, with 1-c cooked asparagus.

I just have to ask. Did you ever have cravings?

Sure I did. My craving was for sourdough toast. Not just the bread. It had to be toasted with butter and/or cheese. As I would stand in my kitchen, taking that first ever-so-delicious bite, I asked myself a dozen times: *"What is in this toast that makes me feel soooo damn good?"* Seriously, I was truly amazed at how quickly my mood lifted, as I ate this treat. I could literally feel my body and mind relax, almost like a drug. I felt so calm. I swear I could have lived on sourdough toast, along with, of course, a few fat/protein drinks.

Did you gain weight from this habit?

I definitely felt my pants get a bit tighter based on how many pieces I ate. If and when this happened, I simply worked out harder, and got back to eating healthier. Ironically, this is exactly *why* I came to believe I wasn't meant to eat. After all, other than a few lousy pieces of toast, I wasn't eating that much, and yet I felt bloated and fat. (I now realize my mind forced me toward this carb due to low serotonin and, thus, perpetuated my cravings, spiked my insulin, caused water retention and all by eating this particular carb.)

And the butter?

The butter, <u>real</u> butter, and cheese, <u>not</u> fat free cheese, were actually a good thing, as they're both healthy fats. As such, they helped lower the blood sugar response caused by the bread.

What do your groceries look like now?

As I write this, I'm having a delicious salad with organic leafy greens, topped with fresh salmon, goat cheese, sea salt, cilantro, EVOO, and fresh lime. Delicious, and so easy to prepare. And no, I do not live on salads. Nor will you have to.

Unfortunately, my kids love junk food. As a parent, what am I supposed to do?

Don't buy it. Don't have it in your house. Why tempt you or your kids with food that you know is unhealthy? Far too many parents use their children as an excuse for why they can't stick to a healthy way of eating. I can't tell you how many times I've heard: "Oh well, you can stay thin, because *you* don't have kids. *I have children!* And they love Happy Meals, hotdogs, Doritos, fries, and ice cream! They want this kind of food! I can't deny them their favorite food!" Sorry, yes you can. With all due respect, this is merely an excuse.

First of all, why would you want your kids to eat this junk food to begin with? It's only a matter of time before they, too, end up with weight issues. You'll also be wondering why they're so moody, depressed, suffering from professed ADD/ADHD, etc. You need to start them on a healthy diet from day one. If not, then please start today. I don't care what they think they want. As their parent, it's your role to try and make sure they eat healthy. As their loving and devoted parent, your responsibility is to avoid buying the carbs that you know are unhealthy. Don't forget, supplements that boost serotonin can easily help you and your children control the cravings for these fat-promoting carbs.

Your thoughts on gastric bypass surgery are what again?

Gastric bypass surgery is, unfortunately, nothing more than a band-aid, a poor one at that, as it only masks the underlying problem. From what I've seen, there are far too many doctors performing this procedure who don't even begin to properly educate their patients on how to avoid putting the weight back on once they leave the operating table. For those who have had this surgery, most continue to eat the same junk food that put the weight on to begin with. I knew a woman who had it done, and, yes, she lost a lot of weight, but her eating habits had not changed in the least bit. She basically lived off a few sips of soda with a handful of chips. You see, her cravings had not gone away, nor did she know *why* she craved this junk food to begin with. So she continued on the same destructive path that got her fat in the first place. With each passing day, she was able to eat just a little bit more. A few more chips. A little more soda. And an extra bite of her oh-so-favorite chocolate cake that faithfully comes calling by day's end. Now does this sound healthy? Of course not. Not only was this woman eating far too little to sustain her bodily functions, but the food she was taking in had absolutely no nutritional value. Furthermore, she may be thinner, but what had she learned to <u>keep it off</u>? Nothing. Unless these patients learn "how and why" their mind keeps forcing them to eat these particular carbs, unless they're able to control their cravings and appetite, this radical attempt to lose weight will inevitably fail.

Based on the obvious misinformation being provided to many of these patients, and realizing my expertise could help this unique area of weight loss, I looked into bariatric surgery centers. Although I already knew that there were doctors and/or aftercare providers who were not properly educating their patients, I was shocked to see just how overweight some of the surgeons and nutrition counselors were. Several needed to lose at least 50 pounds themselves. Yet these are the professed *experts* in charge of helping others lose and maintain long-term weight loss? I'm sorry, but if they can't even do it for themselves, how can they possibly ever help others? As such, I wasn't that surprised when I read their nutritional recommendations. On one website, under FAQs, the patient's question was, "How soon can I drink sodas?" Now, in lieu of responding with, "Sodas are to be avoided, as they're not part of a healthy diet; sodas are nothing but toxic sugar water and harmful to your health; sodas will perpetuate your carbohydrate cravings and spike your insulin, both leading to more fat gain; and sodas will cause mood swings, water retention, etc." But instead of any of one of these excellent health/nutrition tips, their answer was: "Patients should not drink carbonated beverages until at least 3 months post operatively, as the carbonated beverages may cause excessive amounts of gas and balloon the pouch." *That's it?* That's all these experts could offer? Shameful. Even more alarming is that they approved using aspartame, Sweet'N Low, and Splenda. All artificial. All terribly unhealthy.

I must say I find it disturbing, and highly unethical, that the AMA allows this procedure to be done with so little consideration for the long-term care of these desperate, yet trusting, patients. Gastric bypass surgery or otherwise, these insulin-producing carbs will continue to control them. Not only is this an unhealthy, if not dangerous, way to live, but it will also only be a matter of time before their newly designed stomach is stretched out, as before. Not forgetting they will be risking their very life with this surgery. Nevertheless, if you're still serious about having this procedure done, please first read this book thoroughly, so you will at least be better prepared to keep the weight off long after your surgery.

How do you feel about the various weight loss organizations?
Never wanting to speak ill of another, I am, however, here to hopefully educate you so that you can make better choices. That being said, I first and foremost respectfully applaud anyone who at least takes the initiative to try to lose the excess weight. My biggest concern is that after reading their Nutrition Facts Labels, most of their pre-packaged food contains some of the worst ingredients, including aspartame, high-fructose corn syrup, corn syrup, and saccharin. These ingredients will deplete serotonin, thus, perpetuating cravings, weight gain, bloating, and depression. Due to their many harmful side effects, though, weight gain is the very least of your concerns.

My next concern is that one particular diet program has you eating based on points, each food being worth a certain amount of points. Their commercials show their clients blissfully eating such food (AKA: HIGH GI CARBS), as pizza, bagels, desserts, bread, pasta, cereal, etc. This clever marketing strategy is to appeal to those who don't want to live without their comfort food, but they're not healthy choices, nor are they teaching them "why" they crave these carbs to begin with. (I just met a woman on this plan. Her pre-packaged meal was mashed potatoes, mystery meat, and an approved diet soda. I wouldn't have fed that food to my dog.)

By encouraging their clients to eat these processed/refined carbs, they will encourage insulin levels to spike, followed by serotonin levels rising, then falling. At the very least, this program will perpetuate the craving cycle, further fat gain, water retention, mood swings, depression, etc. This diet plan rarely works long-term. If someone is able to lose weight, their first 10 pounds lost will be from water weight. After that, their weight loss will start to plateau. This is because these plans are so often based on low calorie dieting. The bigger problem is that once these people go off the carefully designed, pre-paid eating programs and back to their normal eating habits, they most often will gain all the weight back and more. *Why?* Because once again, the consumer has not learned *why* they have these cravings to begin with, or how they can control them. Without knowing *why* their brain keeps forcing them to consume those insulin-producing carbs, without knowing *why* they are so emotionally attached to these carbs, diet failure is, sadly, inevitable. Another failed diet will lead to a greater sense of failure, which will lead to a deeper state of depression, more weight gain, and with all of this combined, it will surely keep them coming back to these weight loss centers for years to come. Great for their business. Bad for their clients.

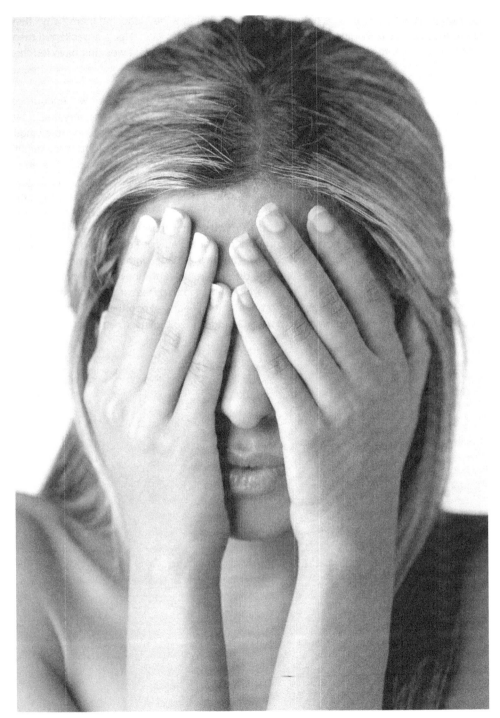

4

THIS IS <u>NOT</u> A DIET

Isn't this just another diet?
No, absolutely not. This is not a diet. Diets don't work. What I'm sharing with you through-out this book is about a "healthy lifestyle." But that lifestyle is completely dependent upon whether or not you can maintain healthy levels of serotonin.

Diets, as we all know only too well, are associated with starvation, deprivation, and frus-tration. Eventually you'll end up with your head in the bag of whatever it is you crave. Cravings will always lead to diet failure. On the other hand, taking a precise supplement that helps safely boost your serotonin, can so easily control your cravings. When you control the cravings, you simply won't have the desire to eat as much, specifically high GI carbs, which spike insulin levels and encourage your body to store fat. You'll no longer eat from emotion. Your professed carb addiction will be gone. You'll eat healthier. You'll eat less. No more binging. All of this will be possible without ever feeling cheated, deprived, or stressed. It will be effortless. I promise you.

Equally as astonishing is that once you maintain healthy serotonin levels, you'll start stabilizing your insulin levels, as well. Your body will then begin to utilize, *to burn its fat stores*, rather than store new fat. Once you truly understand this critical **Serotonin-Insulin Connection,** the secret to long-term fat loss is yours. Never will you have to diet again. You will now know exactly what to do to maintain your ideal body weight.

One of the most powerful aspects of achieving healthy levels of serotonin is that your mind will become quiet—and the cravings will stop. Amazingly, you will then be able to have the carbs you once craved, *the carbs you thought you couldn't live without,* you will be able to have them right in front of you, but you will no longer have the desire for them. Those comfort carbs will no longer have control over you. You will finally be free of the cravings that have always controlled your life and kept you overweight. And that, is exceptionally powerful and empowering.

How does this happen?
To reiterate, once the brain is able to maintain healthy levels of serotonin, it will stop forc-ing you toward the carbs and/or beverages that it used to depend on for this comforting elevation in brain chemistry. Where my clients once thought they couldn't live without their chocolate, sodas, donuts, caffeine, pie, cereal, chips, beer, etc., they now find they simply

no longer have the desire for them. This shift in eating habits is unbelievably subtle. And because of how subtle the changes are, you will need to reflect on just how much your eating habits have changed over time. In addition, there is never any sense of feeling deprived, hungry, or stressed. It is, then, only a matter of time before you lose the excess weight. Adding some sort of weight training will help you reach your weight loss goals even faster. Exercise is a vital piece to a healthy lifestyle.

Never forget that all of this is a process. It takes time. It requires effort. No matter the product, there is no magic pill. Nor will it work overnight, or effectively, if you don't make a conscious effort to eat healthier. With your cravings controlled, it's now up to you to break the old, unhealthy habits. Again, adding some weight training will double your efforts. Sadly, there are many who expect to take a product and wake up with a perfect body. They keep eating the processed junk food that put the fat on in the first place. They continue to drink their daily caffeine, sodas, fruit juice, cocktails, etc., and yet wonder *why* they aren't losing the weight. All these things negate what any such product is trying to help them overcome. Once again, you must be willing to make the effort.

But aren't most people looking for that magic pill?
This is exactly what most people would love to find. Even though there is no such thing. Unfortunately, this truth doesn't deter the production of far too many fat loss products (and weight loss programs) that claim a lean, healthy body can be achieved in "only 48 hours," or by "eating anything and everything you want," or by merely taking a pill at night to wake up thinner. PLEASE! While it is alarming that companies market such useless and often harmful products, it shocks me even more to realize that the consumer actually still believes these products will work.

First of all, the only thing you'll lose in 48 hours is water weight. Secondly, you can never "eat anything and everything" you want and expect to achieve good health. Stop lying to yourself. It is possible, though, by reading this book, to learn how to eat delicious foods such as butter, cheese, eggs, avocado mayo, sour cream, etc., and not gain body fat. It's also possible to lose excess body fat and yet never feel hungry or stressed. All of this—and you will finally understand how to achieve, and maintain a lean, healthy body.

Amazing information! It's all finally starting to make sense. Is this similar to how Fen-Phen worked?
Fen-Phen was an extremely successful pharmaceutical drug treatment for obesity and binge eating disorders. Two drugs, fenfluramine (fen) and phentermine (phen) were taken together, in order to work in what was hoped to be a balanced fashion on two of the body's neurotransmitters: serotonin and dopamine. Phentermine blocked the absorption of dopamine, while fenfluramine worked on blocking the reuptake of serotonin. Fen-Phen made people lose the desire to eat, particularly carbohydrates. It gave people hope. They lost weight like never before. Fen-Phen was the most successful pharmaceutical diet drug

in history. In its prime, drug companies were selling 20 million prescriptions every month. That's about $500,000,000 a month, or $6 billion a year! However, as with all pharmaceutical drugs, it eventually proved to come with life-threatening side effects such as primary pulmonary hypertension and irreversible damage to brain neurons. To reiterate, and I can't possibly say this enough: All pharmaceutical drugs come with harmful side effects, as they alter the "natural" course of the body and mind.

Nonetheless, the medical industry is forever trying to duplicate Fen-Phen's success, minus the horrific side effects. Unethically, doctors were even prescribing the various SSRI (Selective Serotonin Reuptake Inhibitor) antidepressants as not only a way to treat their patients' depression, but also help them lose weight. The FDA finally put a stop to this profitable, highly unethical, if not illegal, practice.

Years later, yet another pharmaceutical drug was introduced to help fight the war on obesity. It's based on elevating the "feel-good" brain chemical, serotonin. *Really?* They're claiming their new diet drug is a "dual-action" product, able to control both carb and nicotine cravings. And, of course, this is true based on the fact serotonin controls both of these cravings. But beware! This is a DRUG! All drugs come with serious health risks. On the other hand, products that are derived from all-natural ingredients (such as those I'm speaking about) can give you the same control minus the above-stated health risks. So I must ask: *Why would anyone choose to take a DRUG that comes with so many serious side effects when you have a variety of dietary supplements that offer a safe, far more effective, and affordable alternative?*

What should I look for when buying a dietary supplement?
Read the supplement panel carefully; review all the claims the product is making; look for precise extracts used, doses of each per serving, quality of the ingredients, amount of product required to be effective, delivery system used to actually get the ingredients into the body, i.e., pills, tablets, gelcaps, or time-release; look for the quality rating, purchase price, and number of servings per bottle (90 days versus 2 weeks). These are all things you should consider before purchasing. Furthermore, if the type on the packaging is too small to read even with glasses, don't buy it. I find it insulting that so many manufacturers use type that is so darn small you can't even begin to read the label. How am I, as the consumer, able to educate myself about their product if I can't read the ingredients or directions, and more importantly—the WARNINGS?

And, finally, for those how may claim they can't afford a $1 per day to maintain their serotonin, well, I'm sorry, but you can't afford NOT to. There's nothing safer or more effective to help you achieve this extraordinary health that I speak of, as there is with maintaining your serotonin with a dietary supplement. Do it for you. Do it for your loved ones. Plus, just think about all the money you'll save from no longer buying all the junk food and having to pay for endless doctor visits and their assorted drugs.

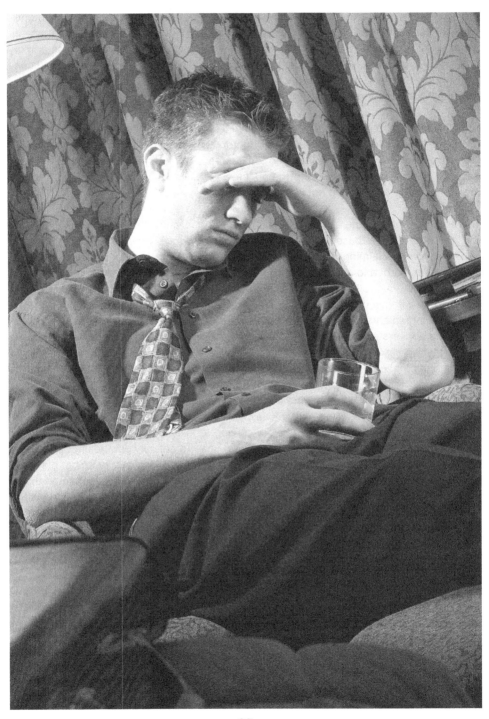

5

HEALTH CONDITIONS ASSOCIATED WITH LOW SEROTONIN

What are the known health conditions related to low levels of serotonin?
Numerous clinical studies reveal that when serotonin levels are low, the following health conditions can arise. As a major neurotransmitter, serotonin regulates so many things within the brain and the body. Therefore, please make sure you do whatever it takes to maintain properly balanced serotonin levels for yourself, your spouse, and your children.

- Aggression (quicker to anger, sudden outbursts, temper tantrums)
- Alcoholism (a physical dependence on alcohol, insatiable alcohol cravings)
- Anxiety (feeling of apprehension, fear, or worry that interferes with life functions) *
- Attention Deficit Disorders (severe difficulty in focusing and maintaining attention)
- Bulimia (binge eating followed by self-induced vomiting)
- Cravings (overwhelming desire for certain carbs, primarily high GI carbs)
- Chronic Pain Disorders (complex chronic pain of joints, muscles, etc.)
- Depression (constant feelings of doom, gloom, inadequacy)
- Epilepsy (brain disorder involving recurrent seizures)
- Headaches (ranging from tension, chronic to migraines)
- Hyperactivity (excessively active)
- Insomnia (the inability to sleep for a duration of time and/or fall asleep)
- Sleep Apnea (caused by a blockage of the airway during sleep)
- Lack of Libido (decreased sexual behavior, ability, desire)
- Mood Swings (extreme changes in mood)
- Myoclonus (brief, involuntary, random muscular contractions)
- Obesity (excess of body fat that is 20% or more over ideal weight)
- Obsessive-Compulsive Disorder (persistent thoughts, ideas, repetitive behavior)
- Panic Attacks (unpredictable attacks of intense fear, discomfort, shortness of breath) *
- Premenstrual Syndrome (symptoms prior to menstruation)
- Schizophrenia (mental illness; mood changes, withdrawn, regressive, bizarre behavior)
- Seasonal Affective Disorder (form of depression/mood disorder with seasonal pattern)
- Suicidal Behavior (actions/thoughts by those contemplating taking their own life)

* Please see page 142: "Humbling Update."

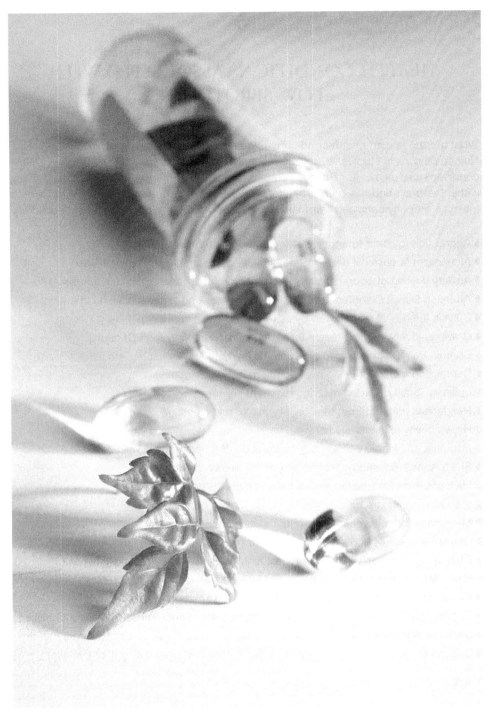

6

HOW TO NATURALLY BOOST SEROTONIN
All natural supplement, no drugs needed

All this talk of serotonin and its many amazing health benefits, but what supplement do you recommend to boost my serotonin?
After several years of researching various extracts, and the subsequent results from having tested those extracts, I suggest the following:

My favorite is the *Griffonia* seed extract, which is rich in 5-hydroxytryptophan, otherwise known, as 5-HTP. This is, after all, the precise extract that I initially read the clinical studies on; the extract that prompted me to spend four years in R&D; the extract that inspired me to spend another two years to write my first edition. Therefore, I highly recommend 5-HTP, a natural amino acid, because it's a clinically proven serotonin precursor. This means it easily crosses the blood-brain barrier (the curtain that separates and protects the brain from the bloodstream) and effectively increases central nervous system synthesis of serotonin. 5-HTP transforms into serotonin once in the body. (Vitamin B6, also called pyridoxine, is suggested to help further facilitate the proper conversion of 5-HTP into serotonin.)

To reiterate, clinical studies have shown that serotonin, the major neurotransmitter that is crucial for both the brain and body to function at their best, also controls cravings, primarily for carbohydrates, and satiety, the body's appetite-control mechanism. Serotonin also promotes mental and emotional well-being, encourages deep restorative sleep, and reduces stress. 5-HTP has clinically proven to be exceptionally effective in treating the dozens of conditions associated with low serotonin. Based on all my research, 5-HTP is, by far, the safest, most effective ingredient to boost serotonin.

Where can I find 5-HTP?
Thankfully, it's inexpensive and available at most drug/health food stores, Amazon, etc. For those with a sensitive system, I recommend "Nature's Best" with an enteric coating. Otherwise, I use NOW or Jarrow brands. You can purchase 5-HTP as is, or as a blend. I highly recommend just the 5-HTP solo. If you buy a blend, do not get one that has any stimulants in it. *Why?* Because stimulants deplete serotonin. They will negate what the product is trying to do, i.e., elevate and maintain healthy levels of serotonin.

Furthermore, 5-HTP is known worldwide as "Nature's Prozac." Unlike antidepressant drugs that come with so many harmful, potentially life-threatening side effects, ranging from nausea, dry mouth, diarrhea, headaches, loss of sex drive, insomnia, to seizures, liver damage/failure, severe withdrawal, depression, suicidal thoughts and suicide—5-HTP can actually help enhance mood, sleep, and libido, while helping to relieve stress, anxiety, and pain. In addition to those many extraordinary health benefits, research from the NCRR (National Center for Radiation Research) found that 5-HTP may also be a powerful antioxidant. The studies suggest that 5-HTP may protect our bodies from free radical formation and oxidative damage, thus slowing the aging process. Wow! *What more can you ask for?* I'll tell you this: If I was ever restricted to taking only one supplement, my choice, *without a doubt*, would be 5-HTP. That is how much value I put on it.

What is the best, most effective way to take 5-HTP?

Unlike so many other supplements, anything that is designed to boost (and maintain) brain chemicals, must be taken on a regular and consistent basis throughout the day. The clinicals for 5-HTP ranged from 50mg/3x daily up to 300mg/3x daily. For maximum effectiveness, it needs to be taken on an empty stomach so it can easily cross the blood-brain barrier. Therefore, please take it 20-30 minutes before your three meals.

Learn how to use the 5-HTP, as *your* life dictates.

MOST EFFECTIVE 5-HTP DOSAGE: Start with the lowest dose of 50mg/3x a day. (Less is *more* when it comes to herbs.) Take your first dose as soon as you get up. Then be sure to eat within 20-30 minutes. Take your second dose before lunch, followed by another before dinner. If you don't eat dinner, take it right before bed. Please make sure you take it on a regular and consistent basis.

Now, as this is merely a beginner dose, after one week, increase your dose to 100mg/3x a day. Same protocol, as above. With this dose, I can easily mitigate nearly any and all cravings for wine, liquor, caffeine, sugar, junk carbs, beer, nicotine, etc. Your mood will also be so much better and you'll be sleeping through the night.

If, however, after two weeks, you find your cravings still aren't controlled, take a closer look at what you're consuming. Remember, if you aren't at least willing to make better choices, including avoiding caffeine, sodas, alcohol, candy, bagels, chips, fast food, cereal, juice, and so forth, you'll negate what the product is trying to do for you. If you have, in fact, been dedicated to eating healthier and your cravings have yet to subside, adjust your dose, adding an extra 100mg for those times when your cravings are the toughest; more than likely, it will be 3p until bedtime. As for myself, and my clients, we do exceptionally well with a range of 100mg-200mg/3x per day. But considering our lives vary from day to day, adjust your dose accordingly to find what works best for "you." You should not need to exceed 300mg/3x a day. The 5-HTP does not affect CNS (central nervous system).

Okay, great! My cravings are indeed far worse late day.

Due to the unlimited factors like stress, caffeine, sugar, high GI carbs, etc., that you'll encounter on any given day, thus, depleting your serotonin, cravings will be worse from late afternoon until bedtime. Be sure to take it three times a day and on an empty stomach.

TO REITERATE: One of the most important things you need to remember is to learn how to use the 5-HTP, as *your* life dictates. One day 100mg/3x daily may be enough. The next, no. Our life, and all the stresses that come with it, change from day to day, week to week. Listen carefully to what your brain is pushing you toward, i.e., bread, candy, wine, pasta, fruit, beer, coffee, etc. Be aware of your shift in sleep and mood, as well. These are all signs of low serotonin. Therefore, up the 5-HTP to 100/100/200 or 100/200/200.

Any other suggested extracts to help boost serotonin?

Although I list a few other extracts below, they come with various concerns. The 5-HTP is, without doubt, the most effective in safely elevating serotonin, without such side effects. * (If you're on an antidepressant, please read page 96, before you start on 5-HTP.)

St. John's wort is a perennial plant. Hypericin, the active substance of this herb, helps to elevate the biochemicals in the brain that affect mood, namely dopamine and serotonin. However, St. John's wort can also elevate norepinephrine. Norepinephrine is classified as an excitatory neurotransmitter. It may cause and/or worsen feelings of anxiety in some people. Please avoid. This is not what you want.

Another, but more expensive option to boost serotonin is SAMe (S-Adenosyl Methionine). It's an amino acid that naturally occurs in the cells of our body. It's known to be essential to at least 35 biochemical processes in the body, including maintaining the structure of cell membranes and balancing serotonin, dopamine, and norepinephrine. SAMe has been successful in treating depression. However, bursts of norepinephrine can lead to euphoria, followed by anxiety, panic attacks, elevated blood pressure, and hyperactivity. Please avoid. This is, again, not what you want.

And finally, noni, a tropical fruit, used successfully for thousands of years by the island people. It's the highest serotonin-binding plant of the Rubiaceae family. Hence, it produces nearly the same health benefits as 5-HTP. Regrettably, it's very limited in clinical studies to support its various claims. Another problem with most noni products is that they're loaded with fruit juice, which equals lots of s-u-g-a-r. Plus, I have no idea how much active ingredient I'm really getting. In addition to the sugar, this, too, is a concern for me.

Please never forget, no matter how phenomenal an extract proves to be, it will only be as effective as the effort you devote to making healthier choices. And, you must be consistent in taking it. Again, 5-HTP is my preferred—and only choice. I have diligently researched, tested, and used this supp for well over 20 years. It allows me to live this healthy lifestyle without effort. I do the same for my clients.

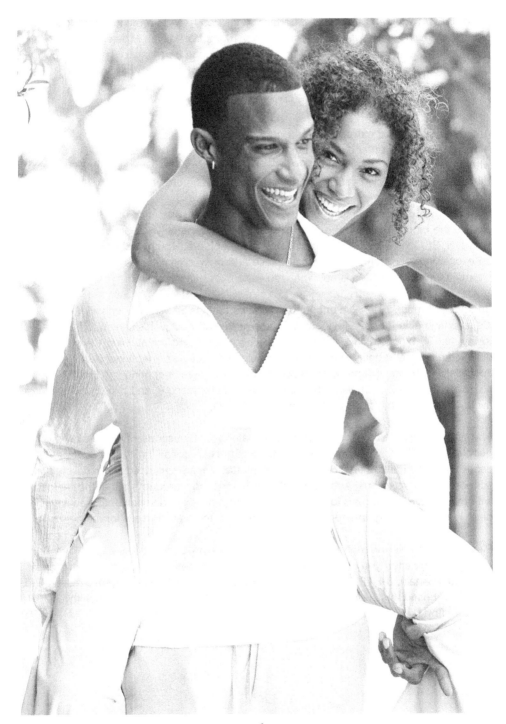

7

THE REMARKABLE
HEALTH BENEFITS OF 5-HTP

How long before I start to feel the benefits from boosting my serotonin?
The many amazing health benefits that will come from enhancing your serotonin will vary in how quickly you actually begin to feel them. The control of your cravings can come as quickly as in one dose, or it may take several days. My clients typically feel the changes in just a couple of days. They're always amazed by how great they feel and how their cravings just went away. Aaaah, glorious serotonin at work.

Once again, the various health benefits do not come all at once. It is a process. It takes time. You must be willing to take any such product on a regular and consistent basis for at least 30 days before making a judgment. (I actually prefer you stay on it for 90 days before drawing any conclusions.) Please keep in mind that the way in which this type of product works, i.e., affecting brain chemistry and without stimulants, is very subtle. But please know this: The longer you stay on the 5 (5-HTP), the *greater* the health benefits.

Furthermore, results will vary tremendously depending on "your" state of health and lifestyle habits. As I stated earlier, if you continue to consume processed carbs, sugar, caffeine, alcohol, etc., you'll negate what the 5 is trying to do for you. Though I consult my clients with regard to what they should eat and drink, it's ultimately up to them. If they choose to ignore me, they must realize each of these factors will greatly affect their progress. While 5-HTP products are formulated precisely to control cravings, you must still put forth an effort. You must be willing to break the old, unhealthy habits. If you keep eating sugar and high GI carbs, even though the cravings are gone, no product will work. This is why I say "effort" is required. You must also realize that if you want a lean, healthy, and attractive body—a body that looks terrific in and out of clothes—you must exercise. Weight training is the most effective way to achieve such a body. The reality is, the key to achieving successful weight loss and overall good health is based on a lifestyle.

Once you realize that this is not a quick fix, but rather a solution, it's up to you what you want to achieve. Is it a sleeker, stronger, sexier body? Would you like to alleviate cravings? Control appetite? Enhance mood? Be happier? Alleviate depression and anxiety? Reduce body aches and pains? Improve concentration and ability to focus? Reduce risk for certain cancers? Diabetes? Stroke? Heart attack and heart disease? Dementia? Alzheimer's? Maybe you have issues with sleep or need more energy? Or maybe you'd like to enhance your libido or slow the aging process? Boosting your serotonin can help you with each of these concerns and more. But because serotonin is depleted by basically everything in life, the key to alleviating these numerous health conditions is to <u>maintain</u> this brain chemical.

Are there any side effects from taking 5-HTP?

There are those who might experience minor nausea and gastrointestinal problems. It's rare and nothing to be alarmed about, as it's simply the 5 getting into their system. It should not be an issue after a few doses. Take enteric coated capsules to help avoid this. Regardless, be sure to eat something healthy within 20 to 30 minutes. Vivid dreams are also possible side effect. This is due to a much deeper state of sleep. For those who claim the 5 can cause drowsiness, I disagree. Drowsiness generally only happens when taking 200mg-300mg at night, come the sleep cycle. My clients may often feel tired, but it's often caused from me weaning them off all the carbs/sugar, caffeine, wine, etc., not from the 5.

Is it safe for children? Both my teenagers could benefit from taking the 5.

Based on the clinical studies; over four years in R&D; plus, my personal experience and that of my many clients—I would say, absolutely. However, the FDA requires supplements to contain a standard warning. Part of that warning states: "Keep away from children." Nonetheless, as their parent, this is your decision. I will say this: If I had a child, I would, without hesitation, have them on the 5.

How much weight can I expect to lose?

This research, along with a quality 5-HTP, is giving you the solution for long-term weight loss. Thus, there is no limit. But, once again, it does not happen overnight. It's not a quick fix or a magic pill. This is a process. It will take time, effort, and commitment on your part. While no such product will ever work overnight, I guarantee you there is no safer, more effective way to achieve your lifelong health and fitness goals of both body and mind than by properly maintaining your serotonin.

How will I know it's working?

You will first feel a huge improvement in your mood and sleep patterns. And then, because the primary actions of the 5 are remarkably subtle, you will slowly, and only in deliberate reflection, look back and suddenly realize how much your eating habits have changed. You will realize how you no longer need that caffeine or soda to get you going. You will no longer miss that chocolate bar that once consumed your every waking thought. No longer will you crave those scrumptious, extra large oatmeal cookies at midday. You will no longer find yourself reaching for the basket of bread or bag of potato chips. No longer will you need that bowl of cereal after dinner to finally feel satisfied. When you drink a soda (diet or otherwise) out of mere habit, it will taste awful and way too sweet. You will be able to go into a restaurant and not want to order everything on the menu. You will effortlessly lose the cravings for those high GI, insulin-producing carbs. You will find yourself wanting to eat healthier food, while also being content with eating less. And *never* will you feel deprived. While cravings and appetite are starting to be controlled, many also feel a huge relief from anxiety, depression gone, and less overall stress. They're much slower to anger. They feel more relaxed, more energized, and a whole lot happier. At the same time, they find their sleep patterns are also greatly improving. All of these things add up to a much healthier body and mind.

Moreover, you will, in all your glory, feel as if you have FINALLY—after all these years of struggling with diets—figured out how to harness and <u>control</u> your addiction, emotional eating, binging, or otherwise. This is because 5-based supps are designed specifically to affect brain chemistry. With your serotonin levels now much healthier, your brain will stop forcing you toward those terribly unhealthy carbs. It's perfectly natural that you will feel like you have finally been able to conquer, to overcome those cravings with pure and simple WILLPOWER. This is why the 5 makes it all seem so wonderfully effortless, because it comes from *within* you. There is absolutely no effort to live a heathier lifestyle, once you are able to achieve and maintain adequate serotonin levels. Again, all of this takes time. It also requires effort to break the old, unhealthy habits. But it will happen, I promise you. Just remember how long it took to get your body (and mind) out of shape. You need to be patient in reaching your goals. Remember, you will lose inches long before you actually lose pounds, so please stay off the scale.

Why don't you want me to weigh myself?
Weigh yourself when starting. Use that number as a marker. Then <u>forget</u> about the scale, as it is not an accurate way to analyze your overall body composition. Furthermore, measuring only your body weight will most often discourage you. Personally, I rarely ever weigh myself. I've learned to not only listen to my body, but also to know exactly where I am, within a few pounds, simply based on how I feel and how my clothes fit. In time, you'll be able to do this, as well. To track your success, measure your waist and insulin gauge, note your weight, more importantly, your body fat, then use those measurements as a guide. For every inch off your tummy, it's worth about 1-2% body fat.

How do I measure my body fat?
Rather than judging your potential heath risks based on the once highly acclaimed BMI (Body Mass Index), a method that does not take into consideration those who weight train and who will, consequently, have more muscle mass, I use a specific device that will test body fat. However, using a measuring tape to track your waistline is a very effective method to measure your overall health. The leaner your tummy, the better. Remember, your waistline is a direct and immediate reflection of how well your diet is working, or not. Whatever the method, don't stress about it. Record the initial measurements and then let it go. Put your full attention on getting healthier.

What is the danger zone for my waistline?
According to the AJCN (American Journal of Clinical Nutrition), anything greater than 40" in men and 35" in women is considered the danger zone. The following chart, though bare minimum, as a healthy level of body fat changes with age, will at least give you an idea of where your body fat should be. There are numerous websites that offer various methods in which to measure your body fat, BMR, EER, etc. I recommend you buy the Omron Body Fat Analyzer (HBF-306C) from bodytronics.com. Just remember, not only are there dozens of ways to test all such data, but the subsequent results, and the preferred healthy numbers, will also vary greatly from person to person depending upon their age, height,

weight, body composition, level of activity, etc.

Body Fat Chart		
Description	Men	Women
Essential fat	2-5%	10-13%
Athletes	6-13%	14-20%
Fitness	14-17%	21-24%
Average	18-24%	25-31%
Obese	25%+	32%+

What does BMR stand for?

BMR (Basal Metabolic Rate) represents the actual number of calories your body needs to sustain your bodily functions without exercise. It accounts for about 75% of total daily energy expenditure. And the more LBM (Lean Body Mass), the *higher* your BMR. The higher your BMR, the higher the rate your body will burn calories/body fat at rest. This is precisely why I keep saying you need to lift weights to build LBM, while also eating properly. LBM will help you not only lose body fat, but also keep it off.

Fascinating! I've never heard of this, but it makes perfect sense. Eat too little, my body goes into starvation mode. Eat too much, it stores the excess as fat.

Very good! While the 5 will control your cravings and appetite, the other crucial key is finding out the amount of fuel your body requires so as to control your weight, more so, your body fat.

I can't wait to get started! Should I stop taking the 5 once I lose the weight?

This is of course up to you, but I would say no, merely because the health benefits of maintaining serotonin goes far beyond just losing excess body fat. The 5 will, yes, help support healthy levels of serotonin, which will, thereby, help control cravings, stabilize insulin, and help reduce appetite. But this is only the beginning. Based on the many extraordinary health benefits that come with boosting serotonin levels, *benefits that are truly life-changing,* I suggest you use the 5 as long as it serves you well. As for me, I take mine eagerly everyday and will continue to do so for the rest of my life.

What happens if I go off the 5? Will my old habits come back?

Allow me to answer that by sharing the following quick story: Because this type of supplement affects brain chemistry, and in such a gentle, subtle manner, it's only natural that my clients suddenly felt as if their newfound willpower was based on them alone. In fact, as I was going through the R&D phase, several of my clients were reluctant to give my product any credit at all. They truly believed that they alone were finally able to conquer their cravings. While I'm thrilled that no matter what they believed was the catalyst in the dramatic change in their eating habits, it was only when they ran out of product that their viewpoint changed.

They were fine for the first few days. But once they were off it for about a week, to their dismay, their old, unhealthy eating habits came creeping back in. Their cravings for cookies, rice, sodas, caffeine, chocolate, corn bread, even cocktails, were suddenly back in full force. Their sleeping patterns suffered greatly. Their moods spiraled downward. They were once again quick to anger, highly irritable, stressed, and, worst of all, they were back to eating the high GI carbs that had always given them such emotional comfort. Those carbs were, unfortunately, the same ones that got them fat and miserable in the first place. They knew it wasn't good, but no matter how hard they tried to control the cravings, they were once again helpless. Their newfound willpower was suddenly gone. My phone began to ring off the hook. My clients were in a panic. They were upset with what was happening to them. They were desperate for more of my product. I hated to see them suffer, but as a product developer—this was all-telling for me. This, unequivocally, confirmed the impressive clinical evidence supporting 5-HTP.

This experience wasn't limited to my clients. You see, throughout R&D, there are untold changes involved in the formulation process. It was inevitable that I'd be without product at times, as I was forever making advances in my formulas. (I expected nothing short of perfection, due to the diet industry being saturated with so many ineffective, over-hyped products.) So, to ensure accurate testing, I periodically went off all ingredients that stimulated my serotonin. I, too, was fine for a few days, maybe even a week without cravings or mood swings. But then, *there it was!* Though my weakness was never for sweets, my craving for a piece of sourdough toast (or dirty martini) suddenly came knocking. Like clockwork, my mind started to force me to consume the things that it once knew would elevate this vital brain chemical. I didn't panic, as I knew exactly why. I, therefore, reflected on my life to see *why* my serotonin would be low. Easy answer: My life is pretty stressed, and stress, as you recall, is one of the primary reasons why serotonin becomes depleted. Plus, I stopped taking the 5. Oh, I couldn't wait to get back on it.

I finally understand why my mood and weight has never been stable. I can't wait to put to use the many things you've taught me!
Nothing gives me more satisfaction than knowing I've inspired someone to live a healthier life. Just remember, though, the 5 will not be as effective, especially lifelong, if you don't truly understand *why* you crave these insulin-producing carbs, or why you're depressed, anxious, always needing meds, etc. Therefore, it was imperative that I first educate others as to this incredible research. Remember, knowledge is power. Knowledge is freedom. Knowledge can save your life. So please, keep reading. *Empower yourself!*

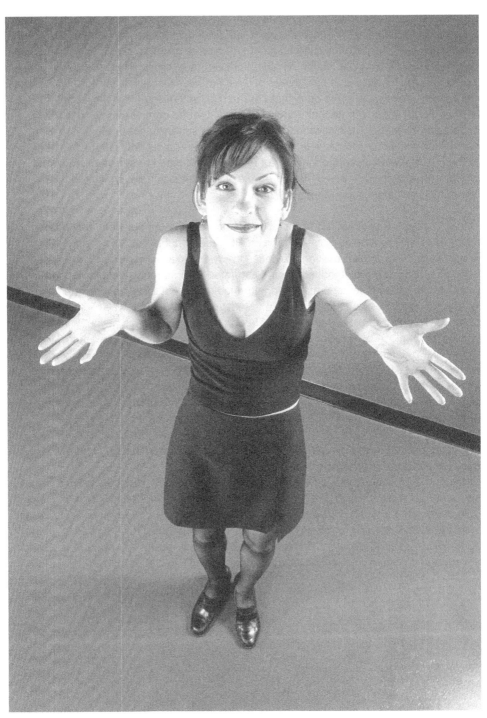

8

UNHEARD OF, BUT WHY?

If what you say is true about serotonin, this information could help millions of people. So why, then, isn't anyone else talking about it?
First of all, it's true and based on sound clinical research, not diet hype. Secondly, if this information was exposed as effectively and with the same intensity as any given block-buster movie, better yet, as the drug companies promote their drugs, it would indeed help millions. Furthermore, there are scientists and a few select health experts talking about it, with excellent books written about it, and most importantly, with impressive clinical studies to support it. Ironically, other than the authors/doctors listed below, I haven't met anyone, be it a doctor, psychiatrist, celebrity trainer, or layman, who was aware of this research. *Why?* Well, for one, less than 2% of all doctors are educated in nutrition. Most admit to getting less than one week of any sort of nutritional training in med school. This is shock-ing, considering most of our diseases are based on nutrition deficiencies. Even the many RDs (Registered Dietitians) and CNs (Clinical Nutritionists) that I've either spoken to, or heard being interviewed, are completely unaware of serotonin.

Speaking of RDs and CNs, I want to share my concerns: I have over 40 years in the fitness industry, specifically the last 22 years devoted to nutrition and neurochemistry alone, but it was while writing this book that I decided to further my education by earning my Sports Nutritionist certification. The rather unsettling aspect for me, however, with regard to the course that is so highly rated by the industry, is that what I'm forced to study and agree with is terribly far from what I know to be true. Their teachings with regard to diet are very old school. And I quote: "There is no good evidence that high insulin levels make people fat." (Liebman, 1996) If that statement isn't alarming enough, most of their research is from the same time period, over two decades old, which clearly explains why they still fear fat. And, as such, they recommend only fat free food (which = too many carbs), avoiding cho-lesterol, i.e., eggs, cheese, butter, etc., while fruit juice, skim milk, nonfat yogurt, cereal, bread, rolls, muffins, pasta, pretzels, bananas, and potatoes are their preferred carb—and primary *protein* sources. Worst of all, they classify Coke and diet soft drinks as "sports drinks," and recommend eating margarine. *They can't be serious?!*

Most athletes believe in carb-loading for quick fuel, but all that sugar is a false and unhealthy way to get energy. Their suggested meals consist mostly of simple and com-plex carbs, but those complex carbs are *refined* carbs. And without any fat and very little protein to help lower the GI, let alone balance the food groups, those declared complex carbs will affect blood sugar levels dramatically and deplete serotonin. For those who work out, those carbs may supply fuel, but if they're not used, they'll be stored as fat. While some may be able to burn off the sugar, the more serious concern is the damage that will be done due to the overload of insulin required to control the sugar. High insulin levels are never good, burned off or otherwise. Even if one still believes in carb-loading, why not <u>low</u> GI carbs? They're far healthier, a more efficient fuel source, i.e., slower burning/longer lasting, and with no insulin spiking. And what about fat? Where's the olive and coconut oils, or avocado? *Our bodies need fat to burn fat.* It's also a far more efficient fuel than carbs/sugar. Moreover, why not eggs or fish as a protein versus "cereal" or "two slices of bread?"

But hey, who am I to doubt their expertise? I mean, after all, they have a "college degree" and I'm merely self-taught. Well, let me just say this: If this 60-year approach to nutrition was correct, if the nutritional advice that the colleges and various health/wellness organizations are passing on to their students is accurate and nutritionally sound (which they then pass on to their clientele), *why* is our obesity rate at 65% and ever-growing? Why are those who are under the care of a CN or RD still struggling with their weight? And, why are the majority of those individuals in the educational/medical positions overweight themselves? It concerns me, because these educators, doctors, etc., will continue to spread this information—and with no end in sight. All the while, what they're teaching with regard to nutrition is going to make the average person gain body fat, <u>not</u> lose it. And, just as I assumed, no mention whatsoever of serotonin by any of these experts. **NEWS FLASH**: On The Today show, an RD recommends, "Diet soda, 6-inch Subway sub, and Lay's Lite Potato Chips for healthy weight loss plan." No comment needed. . .

Now, as for why most consumers are not aware of serotonin, how could they be? After all, if those in charge of educating others are completely unaware of it, how would the typical consumer ever be expected to? This is precisely why I spent the last 20+ years of my life promoting my books with a passionate, and somewhat desperate desire, to bring it to the forefront of society's consciousness. I won't be content until every man, woman, and child is aware of this information.

What prompted you into this area of research?
Through the many years of personal training and teaching my clients nutrition, I watched them frantically try to lose weight with whatever the latest diet craze was. Yet, no matter how good those diets sounded, no matter how many so-called "impressive studies" or raving testimonials they produced, many of my clients were simply unable to control their cravings so as to achieve long-term weight loss. Temporary weight loss was easy. Keeping it off was another matter. All because they couldn't resist certain sinful high GI carbs. My own sporadic craving for toast also astounded me. I knew without a doubt, cravings were something *far beyond* willpower or emotional attachment. Nevertheless, it wasn't until years later when I was a partner in an infomercial project that I shifted my focus from the gym, and went extensively into R&D. The more I learned, the more disgusted I was by the blatant and endless deceit within the diet, food, and pharmaceutical industries.

Where did you actually learn about serotonin?

I've read literally dozens of clinical abstracts, various medical studies, and health journals, but by far the best books I've read on this subject are the following:

5-HTP, The Natural Way to Overcome Depression, Obesity, and Insomnia by Michael Murray, ND, a highly respected naturopathic doctor, best-selling author, and speaker. This book is very detailed and exact, complete with clinical studies to support all such claims, yet it's equally reader friendly. It will reconfirm all that I say about serotonin and 5-HTP, plus much more. I recommend everyone read this book.

The Schwarzbein Principle by Diana Schwarzbein, MD has over 40 years of extensive medical training in endocrinology, biochemistry, and physiology. More importantly, her work is supported by impressive clinical studies. She is an exceptional doctor, as well as respected speaker, radio host, and best-selling author. This celebrated book discusses, among many things, serotonin and cholesterol and their fundamental roles in good health.

"Need more proof?"

However, what I love best is *how* Dr. Schwarzbein came to learn the truth about nutrition. FACT: Most medical doctors do not take any nutrition courses. If they do, it's based on the low fat myth. They are taught fat is bad. Hence, they promote a low fat/high carb diet, which, as you know by now, will create disease. Yet as Dr. Schwarzbein began treating her patients, *and as an endocrinologist,* she discovered the patients who so-called cheated the most on their diet with such things as butter, cheese, eggs, cream, steak, etc., were the ones who were actually becoming *healthier* with each visit. Trigs were dropping, HDL rising, BP stabilizing, body fat and A1c lower—and so much more! She was amazed! But, unlike most other doctors, this doctor actually decided to adjust her way of treating patients based on what she was witnessing. She couldn't possibly keep promoting what she knew was false—and detrimental to her patients. And, out of this, *The Schwarzbein Principle* was born. Extraordinary! If this story doesn't inspire you, I'm not sure what will.

I was fortunate enough to meet Dr. Schwarzbein in 2001 to discuss my research and initial product. I was humbled when she was impressed enough with both, that she considered conducting a private study with some of her patients, while also wanting to private-label my formula. Unfortunately, due to our schedules, it never came to fruition.

The perspectives set forth by the above two doctors with respect to what it takes to achieve overall excellent lifelong health are, undeniably, some of the most accurate of all the experts I've come to know. But, considering I'm a woman who questions everything, clinically proven or otherwise, no amount of clinical studies or books was enough for me. The last thing I would ever want to be part of was another weight loss marketing illusion. Based on the all-encompassing time I dedicated to R&D, the product testing with approximately 50 clients nationwide, along with, of course, my own personal experience, I am confident, *without any hesitation,* in sharing this extraordinary information with you.

All the more reason why I'm shocked to see that not one of the major companies has focused their attention on this remarkable research, subsequently, developing products that would address this essential link. Instead, the diet industry's only focus is forever on using stimulants for weight loss. Considering our obesity rate, that approach is quite obviously not effective. Even though ephedra was pulled from the market, consumers beware: product developers are simply using every other type of stimulant, hoping to promote weight loss. That weight loss, if any, will be terribly unhealthy and short-lived.

My sense of urgency to bring this information to the mainstream also comes from the fact that nearly everyday I hear yet another health expert blaming the public for being "fat because they choose to be, they're too lazy, addicted, lack willpower, no control over their emotions, or they use food to comfort themselves." But to make matters even worse, when you berate someone, when you so cruelly judge them, it only fuels their sense of failure and hopelessness, and deepens their sense of worthlessness. Of course I realize there are always going to be those individuals who are simply unwilling or uninterested in losing weight. Too lazy? Maybe. Confused? More like it. But no one chooses to be fat. No one chooses to fail at every diet they try. No one chooses to comfort themselves every night with a bag of cookies and a liter of soda. No one chooses to be weak-willed. No one chooses to be addicted to anything that would bring them such emotional pain. No one intentionally chooses the many health risks that come with being obese, let alone the unfair public scrutiny.

The fact of the matter is, there are thousands of health experts, telling people a thousand different ways to lose weight (me included). But it's up to you to educate yourself about the various options and determine which ones are based on science, not diet hype. Nonetheless, it's entirely another matter when people, especially people with platforms that reach millions, share their opinions in a hurtful and demeaning manner. It worries me, because with this tremendous power, they can affect millions based on their commentary. I hate to think about just how many people will come to believe they're fat because they're too lazy, without willpower, or they merely, on a subconscious level, *choose to be*. Although I believe these particular people are sincere in wanting to help others, their comments are often brutal and unjustified. No disrespect intended, but I would only hope that those individuals who step into the weight loss arena have the required expertise. At bare minimum, they should equally reflect their expertise via their own physical body. No matter the profession, we should each be able to proudly represent what we expect from others.

I will, though, most certainly agree that people frequently use food to comfort themselves and, likewise, they often seem to lack willpower. No argument there. But it's "why" they eat this comfort food, moreover, why they can't stop using it as a crutch, that most health experts are unaware of. If they were aware of serotonin, the major neurotransmitter that governs cravings, appetite, depression, etc., I'm quite sure they would never make such insensitive comments.

I've heard quite a few people claim that diet failure is due to being lazy, weak-willed, and so forth. I struggled with this, because I was successful in every other part of my life, but failed miserably when it came to sticking to a diet.

You and a million others. Bottom line, no matter how many times or in how many ways anyone, be it Dr. Sears (the Zone), Dr. Agatston (South Beach Diet), Dr. Atkins, or even Dr. Phil, tells you to stop eating processed/junk food or other high GI carbs, it is entirely another matter to actually *adhere* to that diet regime. Statistics don't lie: 98% of all diets fail. They fail because of cravings. *The crucial link to lifelong weight loss is being able to achieve and maintain healthy levels of serotonin.*

I read Dr. Atkins' latest book, and he never mentioned serotonin. I often heard him say cravings were about people being addicted to certain carbs.

You're exactly right. As I read Atkins' 2002 revised book, I was amazed to discover that he, too, was unacquainted with serotonin and its role in successful weight loss. Based on his books and numerous interviews, his expert opinion was that cravings were directly related to "individual food intolerances/allergies or a drop in blood sugar." He also claimed cravings were caused by being "addicted to certain carbs/beverages." Due to his own admission that he couldn't control his patients' cravings, I knew he was unaware of the serotonin-insulin research. It was in January 2003 that I decided to write him a letter. Within weeks, ANI's (Atkins Nutritionals, Inc.) VP of Business Development called. They were eager to talk to me. Regardless, and to quickly summarize: After the pain-staking process of ensuring their non-disclosure/non-compete documents were going to protect me, I signed. I then promptly offered to fly to New York. I knew it was necessary that I speak directly to Dr. Atkins. But I was told he was "not involved in the day-to-day business of ANI." Ah, the corporate veil. The first red flag. My only option was to disclose to an ANI senior VP. Only *after* I reconfirmed with her that Atkins/ANI was indeed unaware of this research, did I agree to move ahead. This hour-long disclosure went so well, in fact, that she expressed interest in ANI private-labeling my formula. But first, she requested I send a copy of my clinical studies and my formula ASAP. I agreed to a partial submission of the clinicals only.

You must have been thrilled to see where this opportunity would take you!

Yes, absolutely. But, to my dismay, only days after the Atkins group received my research, my phone calls and emails were no longer returned. The VP I had dealt with was suddenly nowhere to be found. I'm far from a pessimist, but I knew these signs only too well. When I was finally able to reach her, she apologized for not getting back to me sooner and then claimed, "I'm sorry, but there has been a slight mistake. Dr. Atkins has long been aware of this research. He simply chose not to 'publish' it at this time. We are, nonetheless, still interested in possibly private-labeling your formula."

Without wanting to air any more dirty laundry, let's just say I felt it was in my best interest, and that of my company, to sever any and all negotiations.

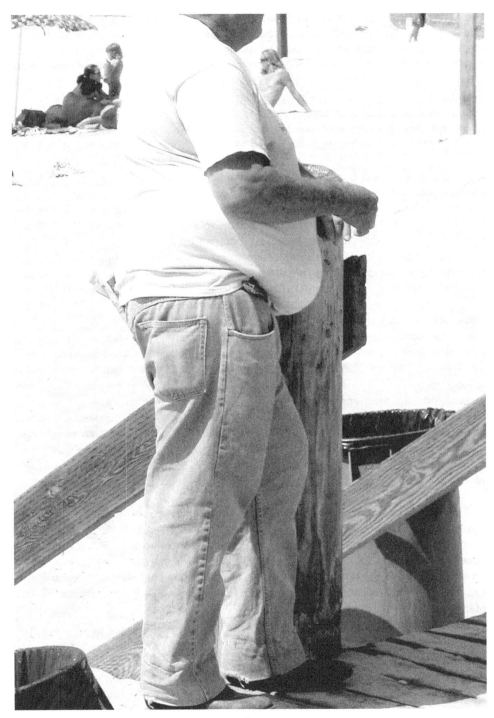

9

STORING BODY FAT
One of insulin's many roles

You've mentioned insulin numerous times, but what is its role?
Insulin is an extremely important hormone, secreted from the pancreas, that lowers blood sugar levels and builds and stores fat. Insulin tightly regulates the amount of sugar going to the brain. It is responsible for putting nutrients (fat, sugar, protein) into cells. Insulin regulates how much blood sugar (glucose, which is energy for the cells) will be allowed to enter the cells. Without insulin, blood sugar rises to harmful levels.

What happens when insulin is released quickly?
Among many things, the rapid release of insulin stimulates the production of serotonin, which makes us feel good, temporarily. This change in mood is so subtle that we are not *consciously* aware of it. The subconscious desire to feel good causes people to eat more carbohydrates. That same desire causes people to eat more food than necessary, which leads to weight gain. It's simple: Low serotonin causes us to eat the wrong food (carbs), and too much of them. Excess carbs need to be used as energy, or they will be encouraged to be stored as body fat, to be used at a later date.

Where does all this sugar come from?
For the last several decades, the American diet has been far too high in carbohydrates, primarily processed and refined carbs, which means *too much sugar*. In addition, numerous types of sugar are hidden in thousands of food items. As we age, the body's metabolic system naturally slows down. The energy that carbs provide are consequently diminished, yet our eating habits do not reflect this change.

Insulin is the garage door opener to our billions of fat cells.

What role does insulin play with regard to fat storage?
Insulin is the fat-building/fat-storing hormone. FACT: Fat cannot be stored on the body without the presence of insulin. Therefore, eating healthy fat cannot cause the body to store fat, because it doesn't trigger insulin. Insulin is the trigger that opens fat cells. Once fat cells are opened, they're like hungry little Pacmen, ready to feed, to gorge, to fill up. Furthermore, once insulin is spiked, it will put the body into a fat-storing mode for several hours. Not only is the body now storing new fat, it will not allow stored fat to be burned as fuel. Once insulin is spiked, by caffeine, stress, high GI carbs, sugar, alcohol, etc., it encourages the storage of body fat from *whatever* nutrient group you eat. Controlling insulin is, therefore, vital to achieving successful lifelong weight loss.

Are you saying that once I trigger insulin, no matter how healthy I'm eating, that food might be encouraged to be stored as fat?
Exactly. This is why you have to be very aware of what you're eating and drinking. Example: Having coffee with your otherwise healthy breakfast will trigger your insulin. *Why?* Caffeine is a stimulant. Stimulants spike insulin levels. Stimulants can also cause insulin resistance. (Let's not forget, that most people rarely drink their coffee black; they add either sugar, nonfat milk, flavored creamer, or artificial sweeteners, all of which spike insulin.) Or maybe you have a chicken breast with white bread, or a side of white rice, with an iced tea. The white bread and rice are both high GI carbs, and both are recognized as sugar by the body. Plus, the iced tea with caffeine. Either scenario has the same result: If you spike your insulin, there is a much greater chance that this food will be stored as fat. Your body will also stay in this fat-storing mode for about two hours.

What else causes insulin to rise?
In addition to the many items listed above, excessive carbohydrate consumption, high-fructose corn syrup, dieting, fat free/low fat diets, stress, prescription and nonprescription drugs, processed and refined food, nicotine, steroids, alcohol, candy, sodas, fruit juices, flavored drinks, iced tea, and lack of exercise will all cause insulin levels to rise.

Sounds like basically everything can spike it. But don't we need insulin?
Sure we do. Insulin makes sure our cells receive blood sugar (glucose) necessary to sustain life. It also increases glycogen storage which provides fuel for our muscles. Nevertheless, high levels of insulin also cause the body to use carbs for fuel instead of utilizing the body's stored fat. Once again, the key to lifelong fat loss, *and numerous other health issues*, is to stabilize insulin levels.

Can increased levels of insulin be harmful?
High levels of insulin over a long period of time are extremely detrimental to your health. Increased insulin can cause fat gain by encouraging the storage of fat, and further weight gain due to salt and water retention. Continuous high levels of insulin cause abnormal and harmful cholesterol production, which leads to plaquing of the arteries. Plaquing of the arteries is the cause of heart disease, heart attacks, and stroke. The over-production of insulin causes insulin resistance, which can lead to diabetes. It also causes high blood pressure, cancer, even death.

What is insulin resistance?
Years of excessive consumption of sugar start to take their toll on our cells. As cells become filled with sugar, they're unable to let any more in. To protect against any additional sugar overload, cells reduce the actual number of insulin receptor doors. Insulin is no longer able to unload as much sugar into the cells. Hence, *insulin resistance*.

WARNING: The fat we carry around our midsection is a pretty good indicator of insulin resistance. This type of stored body fat is considered the most harmful to our health.

Why is belly fat more harmful?

First of all, belly fat is closest to your vital organs. It puts excess pressure on these organs. Researchers believe the culprit is visceral fat, and excess inches around the waist often suggest the presence of visceral fat. This fat contains more metabolically active fat cells. This is in contrast to subcutaneous fat, which is directly under the skin. Visceral fat is more active, releasing toxins into the body. In addition, its secretions go straight to the liver and may interfere with its functions, which include helping to regulate blood glucose and cholesterol. Anyone with a belly has visceral fat. The more you have, the worse off you are.

A recent study published in the *New England Journal of Medicine* gave further support to the notion that visceral fat is more of a threat than fat found just under the skin. Doctors found that liposuction, which removes only subcutaneous fat, amazingly had no affect whatsoever on health, even when surgeons sucked out 20 pounds of subcutaneous abdominal fat. But a person who loses that much weight through dieting and exercise sees significant changes in blood pressure, cholesterol, and insulin resistance.

If you're triggering your insulin, you're not burning body fat.

Liposuction may fail to improve health for another reason. While liposuction removes billions of fat cells, it does not shrink the billions more left behind. Obese people have huge fat cells, with 50 to 75% more mass than fat cells in lean people. Large fat cells are not a good thing to have, because researchers have found that they are more active metabolically than small ones, and more likely to produce harmful substances.

What do you suggest?

The best way to get rid of excess body fat, visceral or otherwise, and shrink fat cells, is through proper eating habits and regular exercise. To reiterate, there is no magic pill or cosmetic procedure that will deliver lifelong results when it comes to getting the lean, healthy, and attractive body that you desire. You have to be willing to make the effort through a healthy lifestyle. You can reach all your goals if you simply come to understand it is about the choices you make, and about being able to control your cravings and appetite. This is also a journey. One that you should enjoy along the way.

IN SUMMARY: Insulin, though needed, is the culprit behind most of our common diseases; obesity, type 2 diabetes, hypertension, heart disease, stroke, heart attack, dementia, Alzheimer's, inflammation, abnormal cholesterol panels, cancer, and so much more. Please, learn how to stabilize your serotonin with the 5, along with reading my book, so you can learn what's truly healthy to eat.

SCIENCE BASED FACTS: Less cravings for junk food/drink, equals less insulin. Less insulin, equals reducing your risks for various diseases. Discover the truly remarkable physical and mental health benefits that come from the *Serotonin-Insulin Connection.*

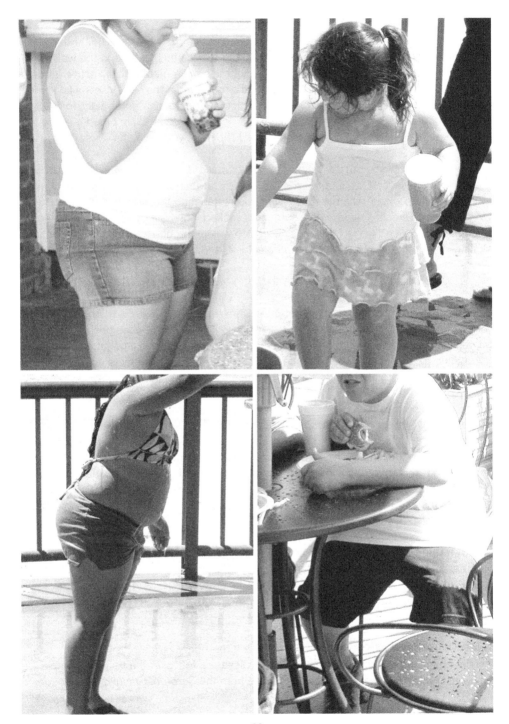

10

TYPE 2 DIABETES RUNNING RAMPANT
Self-induced, yet so easy to reverse

What is type 2 diabetes?
In trying to overcome the cell resistance to excess sugar, the pancreas secretes even more insulin. This causes too much insulin in the bloodstream. The cells react by shutting even more receptor doors. At this point, any sugar in the bloodstream is directed into fat storage. When the fat cells become impacted, the sugar is no longer allowed to enter the cells. It remains in the bloodstream. Hence, type 2 diabetes. Yet, it is so easy to reverse.

Easy to reverse? I never heard my doctor say that.
Yes, type 2 is all about d-i-e-t. I easily reverse this disease for my clients by merely changing their nutrition and lifestyle habits. Learn to maintain your serotonin, and you will, subsequently, stabilize your insulin levels. This will help prevent, and reverse, type 2 diabetes.

What factors lead to diabetes?
The overwhelming number of those being diagnosed with diabetes is fueled by various factors, primarily being overweight. Poor diet, lack of exercise, smoking, and alcohol also contribute to this disease. To lower your risks, a significant change in lifestyle must be made. Instead of the AMA or FDA looking to reduce and even eliminate the *underlying causes* of diabetes, the actual treatment of diabetes has become a billion-dollar industry. But please understand, treating diabetes does NOT cure diabetes. Most treatments may extend life and possibly postpone many of the health issues associated with the disease, but diabetes itself will ultimately take its toll.

Why are so many people becoming diabetic?
This recent surge in diabetes is due to poor diet and lack of exercise. Some interesting facts to consider: A poor diet is due to the inability to adhere to a healthy diet. The inability to adhere to a healthy diet is due to insatiable cravings. Insatiable cravings are due to low serotonin. Lack of exercise is due to simply being too tired, unwilling, or too overweight, which are all due, once again, to poor diet. All of these elements play off of one another.

When serotonin levels are depleted, no amount of willpower or motivation in the world will overcome carbohydrate cravings. For most, the only relief is to consume the carbs and/ or beverages that trigger the quick release of this brain chemical. Unfortunately, the same food (and beverages) that increase the production of serotonin, equally trigger insulin. And insulin is the hormone that causes your body to store fat. Don't forget, this is all occurring on a *subconscious* level. You see, most people really have no idea why they find them-selves grabbing a bag of potato chips and an ice cold soda, or why they're suddenly at the drive-through window ordering a double order of fries, jumbo soda, Quarter Pounder, and a couple of chocolate chip cookies for dessert. From their perspective, it simply sounds *soooo* delicious! They also know only too well just how good this type of food makes them feel! At least temporarily.

No matter how hard you try, *dieting never works!*

While you consume this food, your level of comfort skyrockets. *Ahhhh,* suddenly you feel so good, so relaxed. But BEWARE. At the very same time, your fat cells are gorging. They were triggered open by the spike in insulin caused by this food. Your billions of fat cells are now open wide and feeding. They will remain open and ready to store new fat from any food source, *no matter how healthy it is*, for about two hours after the meal. Your body will also not release any stored fat during this time.

As your serotonin levels begin to drop (and they most certainly will), so will the feeling of emotional comfort you just derived from those carbs. Your energy will plummet. Your mood will do likewise. You'll become aggravated. Quick to anger. Stressed. Anxious. Your brain will then begin the cycle all over again, creating noise, i.e., *cravings* for the type of carbs and/or beverages that it knows will once again trigger the production of this won-derful, mood-altering brain chemical. This cycle is repeated over and over and over again. This is exactly <u>why</u> we have so many new cases of diabetes in adults and, sadly, even young children. Just take a look around. No matter the age or race, everyone seems to be overweight, if not, obese. Those who are in shape are becoming a rarity.

We must also never forget the feelings, the *emotions* that are attached to these weight loss struggles. The feelings of guilt, shame, the total loss of self-respect when you fail at another diet. These deep-seated and complicated emotions further exacerbate the rate of diet failure. You feel even more out of control. Your mood sinks deeper. You feel worthless, hopeless, and alone. No matter how hard you try, *dieting never works!*

But <u>why</u> is it so hard to lose weight, to control the cravings? Are you that weak? Do you not have any willpower whatsoever? You struggle. You cry. Desperate for relief, you eat some candy. With each bite of chocolate, your mood becomes lighter. Bite, after delicious bite, you almost feel normal. Not surprisingly, you eat the entire box. *Ooooh, my!* Relief has finally come! As comforting as it is, you know it's merely a temporary fix. That's okay. You'll take it. For now, it calms your mind. The vicious cycle you know only too well will, however, repeat within a few short hours. You say to yourself: "To hell with it! Tomorrow is another day. I'll start my diet then!" Or you may say, "Hey, I can eat all I want and then just throw it up!" With that, you rush to pick up the phone. "Hello, Pizza King....." (Note: Binging and purging are both symptoms of low serotonin.)

54

Is this why I eat when I'm upset?

The underlying causes of emotional eating can be limitless. But if you are at least able to maintain healthy levels of serotonin, you'll be far stronger, *far better prepared emotionally and mentally,* to deal with these emotional issues. When this happens, it will, subsequently, help alleviate the often overwhelming sense of anxiety, depression, etc., that initially fueled your cravings for junk food, and equally deepened your sense of worthlessness. Until you understand this critical link between serotonin and insulin, this vicious cycle of mood swings, depression, and "emotional eating" will control you. And because serotonin is so easily depleted—causing, at the very least, anxiety, binge eating, and yes, *highly emotional behavior*—your brain will continually compel you toward the food it has long known will elevate it. And, trust me, your willpower is no match for your brain when it wants to maintain this major neurotransmitter. Since high GI carbs are one of the quickest, easiest ways to elevate it, your brain will start the noise, i.e., cravings, for them. You helplessly succumb to the cravings, only to experience once again that overpowering sense of failure. FACT: To control the emotional eating episodes, you must maintain healthy serotonin levels. Once this is achieved, you'll be astonished by how you will no longer seek carbs to comfort yourself. The emotional eating will be controlled. I promise you.

The stomach represents disease. Leaner = reduced health risks.

I finally get it! I really do! But how will I know if I'm eating too much sugar?

To reiterate, the weight you carry around your midsection is the first sign of insulin resistance. It is the first indication that you're consuming more sugar/high GI carbs than your body can utilize. Funny, as their personal trainer and nutritionist, my clients have often tried to convince me they're eating healthy. Sorry. Little do they know that all I have to do is look at their stomach to make this judgment. Their stomach is, again, the most efficient way for me to analyze their diet.

As much as some may honestly try to lose the excess weight, statistics don't lie: 98% of all diets fail. They fail because of cravings. This is because so many things in our day-to-day life deplete serotonin. Maintaining your serotonin is crucial to controlling cravings. Controlling cravings is absolutely crucial to stabilizing insulin levels. Until this is achieved, obesity and type 2 diabetes will continue to rise at alarming rates. (Testing your glucose levels after meals is a great way to monitor and reduce your risk for type 2.)

UPDATE: I've helped numerous clients reverse their type 2 diabetes. So easy to do and just with the 5 and proper nutrition. I reversed one client's diabetes, taking his blood sugar levels from a shocking 397 to 88 in less than a week. His A1c from 12 to 6.9. A doctor heard about my work, asked me to help him with his diabetes. He was able to cut his insulin in half. I also stabilized the blood sugar levels of a type 1 diabetic. FACT: Type 2 is reversible. It's not something you have to live with, or die early from. Have hope and make the effort to live healthy.

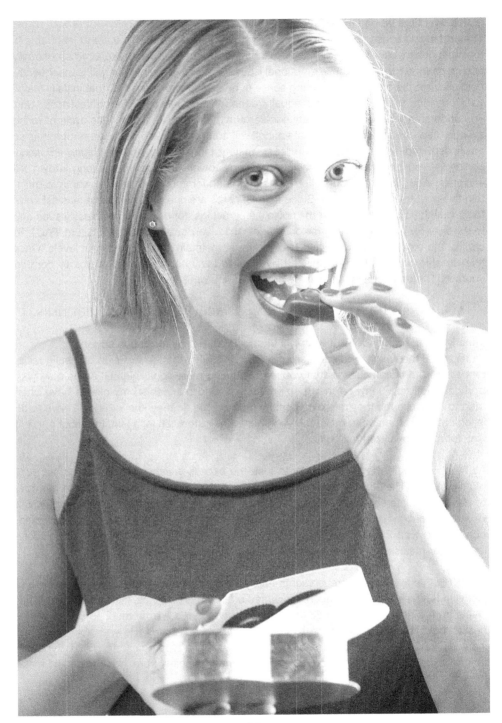

11

SUGAR & ITS HIGHLY ADDICTIVE NATURE
Stronger than any street drug

How did sugar even come into our diet?
The junk-food industry got its start back in the late 1800s. Sugar intake was pretty low to start, averaging a mere 12 pounds a year per person. Suddenly, by 1928, the consumption of sugar was over 10 times that amount. As of today, Americans, on average, consume over 100 pounds of refined sugar per year, per person.

No disrespect intended, but don't believe that you're not one of these people. I say this, because I'm not talking about the kind of sugar you take out of a sugar bowl or even the little packets of sugar. I'm speaking of the sugar that is <u>hidden</u> in over 90% of all processed food, worse yet, in so many professed health products. Sugar is *disguised* under various names in thousands of products. High-sugar products are extremely successful in the marketplace, and they're some of the cheapest fillers in processed food. Sugar is everywhere, from fruit juice, flavored water, vitamins/supps, protein powders, protein bars, sodas, crackers, bread, soups, desserts, baby food, processed food, and canned food. Of course, all those fat free/low fat food are LOADED with sugar. The list is truly endless. So please read the Nutrition Facts and Ingredient Labels with the greatest of care.

Not only does sugar <u>not</u> have any nutritional value, but it's also tremendously harmful to your health. Sugar is a poison to our bodies. It's highly addictive, and there are hundreds of clinical studies that prove just how harmful its affects can be. Sugar damages the immune system, promotes vitamin and mineral deficiencies, not to mention it drains our body's energy. Sugar ages us faster than ever. Personally, I have never experienced anything as addictive or harmful for the mind and body as sugar. Perfect scenario: My close friend Billy always likes to give me a box of decadent truffles for Christmas. And while I don't have any cravings for sweets, I plead with him each year to *pleeeease* not give them to me, as even I, at certain times, can be seduced into eating them. Now there are those who can enjoy one and that's it. But not me. Once I take that first glorious bite, my mind is immediately triggered by the sugar, and it keeps forcing me to eat more. I have even gone as far as to put them in the freezer so it wouldn't be as easy to eat them. Yeah, right! *Who was I kidding?!* Instead, I would find myself taking one, slowly nibbling on it, and then simply letting it melt in the warmth of my mouth. *Oooooh!* Talk about sinful! Hmmmm!

However, as delicious as it may have tasted, the problem was that only minutes after eating it my brain would create that noise, that ever-nagging little voice, that voice we now know is a craving. As hard as I tried to ignore it, it would keep at me, whispering over and over again, "Pssssttt hey—those truffles are in the freezer just waiting to be eaten! Have one more! Come on! That's all. *Just...one...more!*" So I'd have another. And another. And then—one more. Talk about addictive. Once again, I say: I have never experienced anything as addictive as sugar. Since then, if Billy gifts me with those chocolate delights, I take only one, savor its sweetness, and then I quickly, and with great precision, whip the rest of them down the hillside.

Beyond the addictive aspect, sugar damages the body by causing hypoglycemic reaction (low blood sugar). Sugar is actually more toxic than alcohol. It was once written in a Harvard health journal that if "Sugar was just now coming out, the FDA would classify it as a drug." It should at least come with WARNING labels.

NEWS FLASH: Researchers from Princeton announce, "Sugar is as addictive as cocaine and heroin." Amazing, they report this like it's breaking news.

Didn't they add some silly sugar tax a couple years ago to help prevent obesity?
With regard to the two-cent "sugar tax" placed on soda/juice/candy, with intentions of diminishing obesity in children, I found this absurd. Do they really believe that an additional two cents tagged onto these items will deter kids from buying them? Of course not. The thought process behind this tax increase is, in itself, childish, as well as, useless. First of all, the FDA should heavily fine the companies who manufacture this type of food, as it's not a secret that these companies will do whatever it takes to keep the consumer buying their particular products. And the best way to ensure that the consumer keeps coming back for more is to get them *addicted* to their products.

The FDA and FTC should go after those companies with a vengeance, particularly those who *knowingly* practice deceitful/fraudulent marketing tactics. But rather than going after the source, they disturbingly allow these huge money machines to keep putting out this junk food, getting a vast majority addicted, which most certainly contributes to the alarming rate of obesity, heart disease, cancer, depression, etc. And then, on top of that, they want to further tax these food items? *This is wrong!* It is not the government's place to try to control what we eat, through taxation or otherwise, especially considering they knew this food was unhealthy and addictive to begin with. A tax will not solve anything. A disturbing pattern: Cigarettes, knowing full well they were addictive and deadly, but allowing them to be marketed. Then charging those who used them higher taxes. A perfect marketing plan, as the government knows these people are long addicted, and will therefore pay whatever the asking price. Never forget: They also realize the exorbitant amount of profit involved in treating the diseases associated with smoking and obesity. There are far too many people, who make far too much money, to ever put an end to selling these types of harmful products, or their deceitful marketing practices. As of the Vioxx scandal in 2004, the FDA is most assuredly one of those making billions off this deception.

I want to share a rather enlightening comment made by Ricky Williams, the NFL football payer who unexpectedly resigned years back. Mike Wallace was interviewing him on *60 Minutes*. Mr. Wallace, with his usual flair, asked Ricky if he was using any other "more dangerous drugs" than his admitted marijuana. Ricky looked intently at Mr. Wallace, pondered his question, and responded with extreme clarity, "Do I use anything *more dangerous*? Hmm, yes, I suppose I do." (Camera quickly cut to Mr. Wallace with this look of astonishment!) Ricky continued by saying, "Yes, I occasionally eat sugar, as in sweets." Mr. Wallace was dumbfounded by this comment, but I thought it was *absolutely brilliant*. Good for you, Ricky. I admire you for following your heart when it concerned your career, and for recognizing and calling out where the real dangerous drugs exist: in our food.

What other hidden sugars should I watch for?
The following chapter lists the numerous names under which sugar can be disguised. Although I want you to take the time to familiarize yourself with these various names, so you can avoid them, it will be nearly impossible to avoid sugar or artificial sweeteners all of the time. Just do your best to eliminate them, as much as possible.

Besides the highly addictive nature of sugar, it has also been known to:
- Fuel cancer cells • Cause hormonal imbalance • Contribute to obesity and diabetes
- Cause depression and insomnia • Lead to drinking problems, even alcoholism
- Contribute to osteoporosis, worsen PMS and increase risk for yeast infection
- Promote excessive food consumption in obese people • Cause epileptic seizures
- Promote the death of our cells • Increase harmful production of cholesterol
- Deplete vitamins and minerals • Cause hypoglycemia • Decrease growth hormone
- Cause premature aging • Age our skin by damaging collagen structure
- Slow down the ability of the adrenal glands to function properly
- Cause tooth decay, headaches, migraines, arthritis, and heart disease
- Decrease insulin sensitivity, thereby greatly contributing to obesity
- Increase the systolic blood pressure • Suppress the immune system
- Increase risk of high blood pressure • Cause drowsiness and decrease energy
- Alter the proper absorption of protein • Impair the structure of DNA
- Severely reduce learning ability in children • Contribute to Alzheimer's
- Cause hyperactivity, anxiety, difficulty concentrating, and moodiness
- Promote an increase in triglycerides • Cause a spike in adrenaline

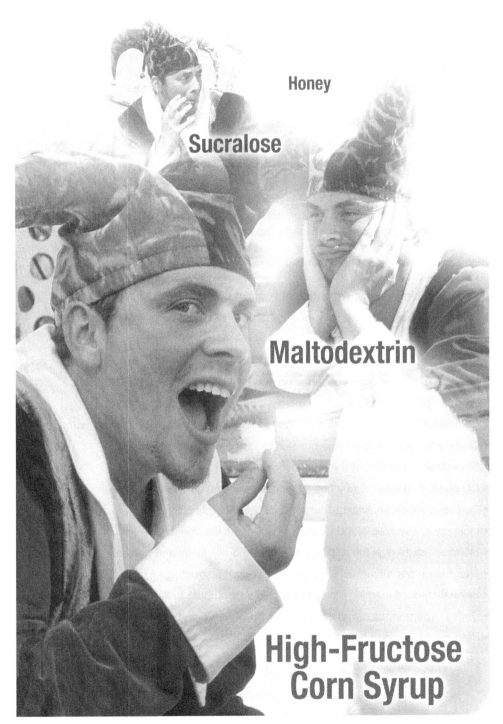

12

THE MANY FACES OF SUGAR

With all this talk of sugar, it's important that you know some of the many different names under which sugar, sugar substitutes, sugar alcohols, and artificial sweeteners are masquerading. Hopefully, this list will help you make better choices when selecting your groceries. Please keep these various names in mind, as you read Ingredient Labels found on food. Please do your best to avoid them.

Types of sugar:

Beet sugar	Brown sugar	Cane sugar/cane juice
Corn sugar	Confectioner's sugar	Corn syrup/corn syrup solids
Granulated sugar	HFCS	Honey
Invert sugar	Isomalt	Maltodextrin
Maple sugar	Maple syrup	Molasses
Raw sugar	Dehydrated cane juice	Date sugar
Glucose solids	Sorghum	Turbinado sugar

Words that end with "ose" are also a form of sugar:

Dextrose	Fructose	Galactose
Glucose	Lactose	Levulose
Maltose	Sucrose	

Words ending in "ol" are yet another form of sugar, known as sugar alcohols:

Maltitol *(used in sugar free food)*	Mannitol	Sorbitol
Erythritol *(used in KETO products)*	Xylitol	Isomalt

Artificial sweeteners:

Cyclamate	Aspartame *(used in sugar free/fat free food)*
Saccharine	Acesulfame-K (aka: Acesulfame potassium)
Neotame	Sucralose *(used in sugar free/fat free food)*

Brand names containing artificial sweeteners:

Equal/Equal-Measure	NutraSweet	Splenda
Spoonful	Sweet N' Low	Sweet One

If you truly want good health—
AVOID SUGAR AND ITS MANY SUBSTITUTES

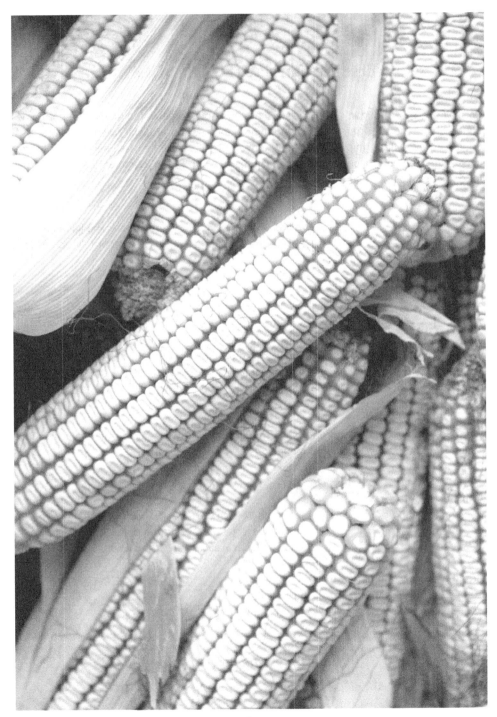

13

WARNING:
HIGH-FRUCTOSE CORN SYRUP

I see high-fructose corn syrup everywhere, but what is it?
High-fructose corn syrup, also known as HFCS, is made from cornstarch. It's a thick liquid that contains two basic sugar building blocks: 55% fructose blended with 45% glucose. HFCS is produced by processing cornstarch to yield glucose, and then processing the glucose to produce a high percentage of fructose. It's basically white cornstarch turned into a crystal clear syrup.

The process for making this sweetener out of corn was developed in the 1970s. The demand for it grew rapidly, from less than three million tons in 1980 to almost 8 million tons in 1995. Consumption of HFCS rose 1,000% between 1970 and 1990. As of 2004, Americans consumed far more HFCS than sugar. The average consumer would be surprised to learn that the larger percentage of sweeteners used in processed food comes from corn, not sugar cane or beets. Sweeteners made from corn account for over 55% of the sweetener market. *Annual sales are over $4 billion!* According to the U.S. Department of Agriculture, consumption of various sweeteners had risen in the United States from an estimated 113 pounds per person in 1966 to 147 pounds in 2001. As for HFCS, we consumed almost 63 pounds per person.

What's the advantage over cane sugar?
There are several advantages of using HFCS. Corn is much cheaper and twice as sweet as refined sugar. As a liquid, HFCS is also easier to blend into various food products, beverages, etc. Food manufacturers prefer it over refined sugar, as they can use less, yet get the same wonderful sweet taste as cane sugar.

Where is HFCS found?
HFCS is laced into *literally thousands* of food products, including chewing gum, pickles, fruit-flavored drinks, cookies, jams, soft drinks, baked goods, fast food, bread, cereal, sauces, bacon, crackers, candy bars, chips, etc. It's basically used in all processed food. Worst of all, it's even found in health products like protein and nutrition bars, dry roasted nuts/seeds, as well as, purported natural fruit drinks and sodas.

How do I know if a product contains this syrup blend?
You need to read the Nutrition Facts Panel, specifically the ingredients section.

Why don't you recommend it?
There are hundreds of studies that show just how unhealthy HFCS is for the body and mind. For starters, it's processed differently in the body than glucose. Glucose causes the pancreas to release insulin. Studies suggest, however, that HFCS does not trigger the release of insulin, nor does it breakdown like glucose. Unlike glucose, where approximately 40% gets metabolized by the liver, HFCS goes directly to the liver. Consequently, the liver converts it far more readily into lipids. Lipids are the chemical building blocks of triglycerides, i.e., fat. (Although the studies I read claim HFCS does not trigger insulin, I disagree. Either way, it's most certainly playing a major role in our obesity epidemic.)

Oh, I am so confused!
Sorry. I know it can be rather hard to follow. Let me simplify it: The body processes HFCS differently than it does old-fashioned cane or beet sugar. It also forces the liver to put more fat in the bloodstream. The end result: Our bodies are basically tricked into wanting to *eat more,* while at the same time we are *storing more* body fat. HFCS also depletes vitamins and minerals, and accelerates the aging process at the cellular level.

Now I get it. I realize now why we're all so damn fat, always hungry, bitchy, and looking older by the minute!
Please don't get discouraged. Simply make sure you read food labels and avoid HFCS, corn syrup, corn syrup solids, and fructose.

I assume these sweeteners will also deplete my serotonin?
Most definitely. These sweeteners will perpetuate cravings and encourage weight gain, mood swings, insomnia, binge eating, depression, heart disease, and so forth.

I'm sorry, but I'm still a little confused. I thought fructose was from fruit, which is healthy, right?
Fructose naturally occurs in both fruit and corn. The fructose I'm talking about here, is made from corn. And high-fructose corn syrup is fructose that has been highly concentrated. Fructose has been aggressively touted for years as a natural sugar. This marketing deception has gone over quite well, considering we've been led to believe since childhood that all fructose comes from "fruit." Hence, it must be healthy. But hold on a minute. Once again, this particular fructose that is being used in our food is not from fruit. It's a refined sugar and harmful to our health. Fructose, corn syrup, and HFCS are large-scale commercialized sweeteners. Eating fruit in its natural form is far different from eating processed food containing fructose, corn syrup, or HFCS.

Understood. I'll make sure to read food (and beverage) labels to avoid buying anything containing fructose, corn syrup, and especially HFCS. Now, can you please tell me once again what triglycerides are?
Triglycerides are the chemical form in which most fat exists in food, as well as in the body and blood plasma. If you eat more carbs than your body can use, the excess are converted

into triglycerides and transported to fat cells to be stored. Hormones regulate the release of triglycerides from fat tissue so they meet the body's specific needs for energy between meals. Elevated triglycerides contribute to heart disease.

Controversial sweetener is banned.

Allow me to close this chapter with a very encouraging news story. Earth Fare, a North Carolina chain of health food supermarkets, has banned all products made with HFCS. Over a third of all their sodas and energy bars will have to be removed, some of them best-sellers. Their plan is to remove all products containing HFCS. This is one of the best stories I've read in a very long time! I applaud Earth Fare for following their mission of "Good Heath," no matter the effect to their profit margins. Most other vendors blindly turn their heads to the numerous health risks associated with HFCS, following, instead, the almighty dollar. This bold stand by Earth Fare also shows just how much they really do care for their customers. As consumers, we should expect the thousands of other retail stores and manufacturers to have the same sense of ethical consciousness.

The Natural Foods Merchandiser reported that Newman's Own has also started to remove HFCS from all their products. Again, great news! Hopefully, this trend will continue.

UPDATE: The HFCS industry has begun to runs ads in attempt to glorify their harmful, addictive product. Among many things, these manipulative ads claim that HFCS is safe, as it's "made from corn, doesn't have artificial ingredients, same calorie count as sugar, and like sugar, fine in moderation." Please do not fall for this self-induced hype.

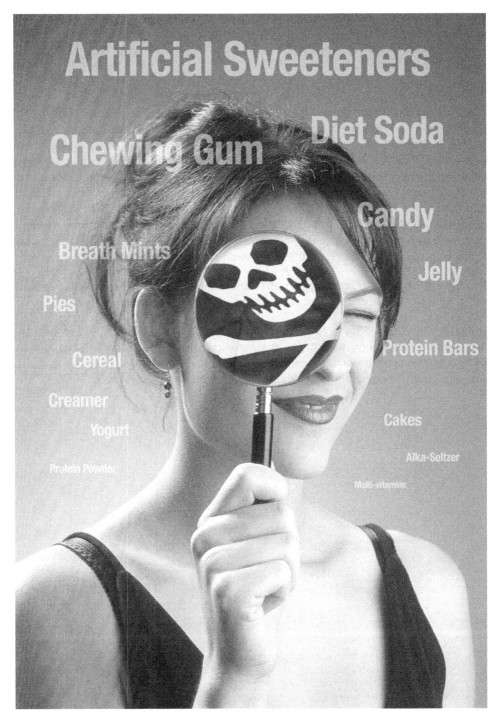

14

ASPARTAME—A DEADLY TOXIN
Making us fat, depressed & deathly ill

To the millions of women (and men) who think they're doing the right thing by drinking diet sodas in lieu of regular sodas, PLEASE STOP. I'm sorry to inform you, but these diet sodas are actually <u>encouraging</u> fat gain, cravings, binge eating, mood swings, anxiety, depression, ADD/ADHD, water retention, and much more.

How's that?
First of all, did you know that diet sodas and most diet food actually *encourage* the storage of body fat? *Why?* Because they're loaded with aspartame, an artificial sweetener. Aspartame is marketed under such names as NutraSweet, Spoonful, and Equal. It is a DEADLY CHEMICAL POISON, disguised as an artificial sweetener. Phenylalanine makes up 50% of aspartame. Phenylalanine is neurotoxic. (Meaning: It damages the nervous system, causing headaches, dizziness, nausea, etc.) Phenylalanine goes directly into the brain, and, at the very least, it depletes serotonin. Phenylalanine can damage neurons in the brain to the point of cellular death. If that isn't enough to scare you away from diet sodas (or diet products in general), diet sodas most often contain caffeine, which will spike insulin levels, thereby further depleting serotonin. You know by now the many serious health risks associated with low serotonin.

Are you serious? Where is aspartame used?
Aspartame is the most commonly used artificial sweetener. The average American consumes over 148 pounds of artificial sweetener each year. Most of it's aspartame.

How can this be? I don't use the stuff that often!
You don't have to use it from a sugar packet. Like HFCS, aspartame is equally prevalent in numerous food products (diet or otherwise), ranging from sodas, cereals, breath mints, chewing gum, candy, protein bars, protein powders, wine coolers, coffee creamers, tea beverages, multi-vitamins, almost all sugar free and lite products, coffee drinks, juice drinks, yogurt, even Alka-Seltzer. If you have products with aspartame in them, throw them away—and do not buy anything ever again that contains this deadly sweetener.

Are you saying my diet soda encourages my food to be stored as fat?
This is exactly what I'm saying. And because every diet soda contains aspartame, women especially need to pay very close attention to this. Little do they realize, as they go about

their day, having an otherwise very healthy lunch of fresh salmon, spinach salad, along with an ice cold diet soda; the diet soda with its aspartame, will actually encourage their food, *no matter how healthy*, to be stored as fat. But after what you just read, weight gain is one of your least concerns.

Oh, my! This is awful! All this time I thought I was doing the right thing!
Yes, you and millions of others. To reiterate, your serotonin will be depleted by the aspartame (and the caffeine), which will perpetuate sugar cravings, weight gain, binge eating, mood swings, bloating, depression, ADD/ADHD, insomnia, decreased sex drive, etc.

Isn't aspartame considered safe?
No. Studies have linked aspartame to *Sudden Death Syndrome.* It's also shown to cause brain tumors, irreversible brain damage, cancer, seizures, depression, suicidal tendencies, aggression, impotence, sexual problems, headaches, migraines, bloating, confusion, hypothyroidism, chronic fatigue, increased heart rate, edema, aspartame addiction and cravings for sweets, menstrual problems, hair loss, chest pains, asthma, vertigo, panic attacks, paresthesia or numbness of the limbs, severe slurring of speech, tremors, difficulty breathing, phobias, memory and vision loss, and much more. At the very least, aspartame depletes serotonin, thereby perpetuating cravings, stimulating appetite, encouraging weight gain and depression.

All of this from an artificial sweetener?
Yes, and there are many more alarming and documented side effects. But don't take my word for it. As with everything I write about, I encourage you to do your own research. See for yourself. Make your own decisions. Believe it or not, it gets worse. Aspartame contains three chemicals: aspartic acid (40% of aspartame), phenylalanine (50% of aspartame), and methanol (10% of aspartame). While both aspartic acid and phenylalanine come with their own serious health risks, methanol is known as wood alcohol, or *methyl alcohol.* Toxic levels of methanol mimics MS (Multiple Sclerosis), ALS, and Lupus, while causing brain swelling, blindness, and inflammation of the pancreas and heart muscle. Aspartame poisoning mimics numerous other diseases. Even more frightening is that, based on the Trocho Study done in 1998, aspartame converts to formaldehyde in those who ingest it. Many of the symptoms reported by victims of aspartame toxicity are undeniably those associated with the poisonous and cumulative effects of formaldehyde.

Why the hell doesn't the FDA pull it from the market?
Why? Money. Greed. Simple as that. Though the FDA has received well over 10,000 aspartame-related complaints, more than all other complaints combined, shockingly it doesn't believe there is any concern, since the substance is used in such small doses. Regardless, the cumulative effects of aspartame are what you should be concerned with. Yet the FDA still considers it "safe." Many believe otherwise. Avoid aspartame at all cost.

This explains why I always feel so bloated and aggravated after I drink my diet soda.

Would I be better off drinking regular sodas?

No, not at all. Regular sodas are nothing more than liquid candy. They're loaded with sugar, caffeine, and chemicals. All of which deplete serotonin. There are caffeine free sodas, but they still contain sugar. Once again, if you drink sugar free, you end up with aspartame (or sucralose).

One of the latest sugar substitutes is Splenda. What are your thoughts on it?

Splenda, the brand name for the non-nutritive sweetener sucralose, is a low calorie sweetener. Of all the sweeteners, sucralose, discovered in 1976, is the only one made from table sugar. Because it's made from sugar, McNeil Nutritionals, the makers of Splenda, claim it tastes like sugar. Studies show it's about 600 times sweeter than sugar and can be used safely in place of sugar to eliminate or reduce calories in a wide variety of products.

How is it made?

It's created by chemically altering sucrose (table/white sugar). In the five-step patented process, three chlorine molecules are added to a sucrose i.e., sugar molecule. And the dangers of chlorine are many. The U.S. Environmental Protection Agency (EPA) has found dioxin, a toxic by-product of chlorine, to be 300,000 times more potent as a carcinogen than DDT.

Furthermore, this type of sugar molecule does not occur in nature. Thus, your body cannot properly metabolize it. As a result of this unique biochemical make-up, McNeil makes it's claim that Splenda is not digested or metabolized by the body, making it have zero calories. But don't be fooled by this claim. The *only* reason it's a zero calorie product is because your body can't metabolize it.

So, I guess the real question: Is Splenda safe?

No, it is not. Only six human clinical trials have been conducted on Splenda, i.e., sucralose. Out of those six minimal trials, only two were finished and published before the FDA approved sucralose for the marketplace, i.e., human consumption. Even more alarming is that the two published trials only used 36 human subjects, with only 23 actually given sucralose for testing. It gets even worse. The trial testing lasted only four days—and the studies primary focus was sucralose and its relation to tooth decay, *not human tolerance*. Furthermore, none of these studies included children or pregnant women.

Nevertheless, according to the far too few studies that have been done, the FDA currently considers it GRAS (Generally Recognized as Safe). As a result, in 1998 they gave it full release to be used in hundreds of food and beverage products. Trust me, this is based on the astronomical profits that will come from this latest sweetener, not because it's safe. As with anything, it takes years of being on the market before a full scope of potential health risks can truly be known. Thus far, pre-approval research showed that sucralose caused shrunken thymus glands (up to 40%) and enlarged liver and kidneys. Based on its chemical structure, it's also possible that after years or decades of use, it may contribute to serious chronic immunological or neurological disorders. My opinion is that anything that is altered chemically is not safe.

Personally, being a woman who doubts most everything, I needed to test Splenda myself. I used one packet in a cup of decaf tea. Within an hour, I found myself with a rash on my neck, and more frightening yet, my vision was dramatically affected. I saw those little back dots and waves of light for nearly 30 minutes afterward ingesting it. Fluke? I seriously doubt it. My body simply being too sensitive? Well, that is a good thing, especially when it comes to poisons. Based on what I've researched, along with what I've experienced firsthand, I will never (knowingly) use Splenda/sucralose again.

Splenda replacing aspartame.

PepsiCo is launching Pepsi One, a diet drink sweetened with Splenda. Their classic Diet Pepsi sweetened with aspartame will still be available. Coca-Cola will also be offering a new diet coke sweetened with Splenda. Likewise, their classic Diet Coke sweetened with aspartame will still be available, as well. To reiterate, sodas are often loaded with caffeine. If they're caffeine-free, they still contain highly questionable and toxic ingredients. I suggest you avoid sodas whether they're diet or regular, or sweetened with Splenda or aspartame.

If not table sugar, aspartame, HFCS, or Splenda, what should I use?
Good question, as it's all a bit confusing. Personally, I would rather use something that is from an herb or a fruit than something that has been chemically altered. While I do my best to avoid all sugars and artificial sweeteners, sometimes it's nearly impossible. Nonetheless, just making yourself aware of the many hidden sugars and sweeteners will help you tremendously in reaching your weight-loss goals.

Stevia: *Stevia Rebaudiana* is an herb in the chrysanthemum family. Stevia is a non-caloric herb, an all-natural sweetener, 300 times sweeter than sugar, and it doesn't affect blood sugar levels. It's been used safely for centuries without side effects. Stevia is extremely sweet, so you need to use very little. There are those who complain of its long aftertaste. I suggest you try using less and trying using a liquid form. Nevertheless, stevia is my favorite sweetener. I believe it should be freely offered in all restaurants, as we deserve a healthier choice. Until that day comes, I carry my own in my purse.

Wisdom Natural Brands, the manufacturers of SweetLeaf Stevia brand, has created a wonderful new line of stevia products called Stevia Clear. These liquid stevia-based products are 100% natural and come in some delicious flavors, including vanilla cream, apricot nectar, chocolate raspberry, English toffee, and many more. You can add them to flavor your water, herbal tea, protein drinks, etc.

WARNING: Beware of similar liquid stevia products, as they may contain grain alcohol, also known as ethyl alcohol. They can also contain glycerin. Avoid these products.

Please never forget: It's also possible to enjoy your food and beverages without using any sweeteners, sugar, or artificial sweeteners. Allow yourself time to adjust to the wonderful flavors found naturally in food.

DIRTY KETO / BEWARE: Some people who promote what I call, dirty KETO, often recommend products/meals that claim they're sugar free. Not true. This food is actually sweetened with erythritol, a sugar alcohol. They eagerly pitch their KETO-friendly pancakes and sugar free syrup to the unsuspecting consumer. First of all, this is nothing more than low serotonin at work. If I crave a pancake, a starchy, crap carb, that is low serotonin. If I crave some sugary syrup, that is most definitely low serotonin. Please avoid these products, recipes, etc. This is not, by any means, healthy or what you want.

Furthermore, erythritol and/or other sugar alcohols, can cause serious side effects from bloating, diarrhea, bloody stools, gas, cramps, headaches, even a possible visit to the ER. The solution here is to stabilize your serotonin so you don't need or want this type of food. Then, please learn what is truly healthy by continuing to read my book. I say in all modesty . . .

Mother Nature's Favorite Sweetener:
Stevia

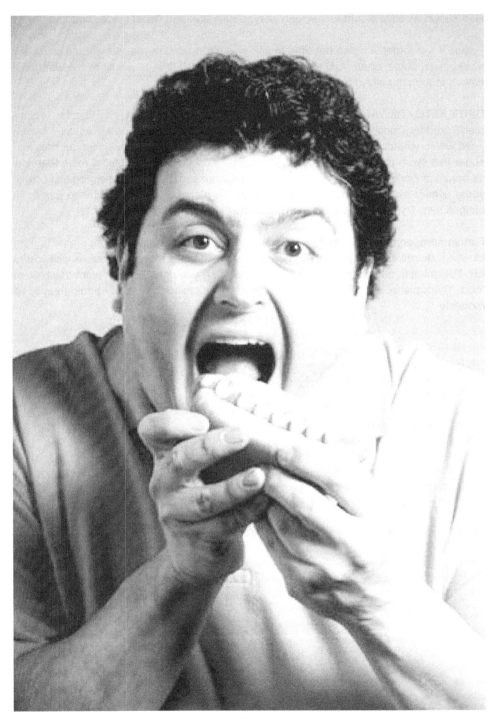

15

OBESITY
An alarming epidemic

First of all, when is a person considered "obese" versus being overweight?
A person would be considered obese when they are 20% above their ideal weight for age, height, and bone structure.

What about pertaining to body fat?
A woman is considered obese when her body fat is 32% and higher. A man is considered obese when his body fat is 25% and higher.

Isn't obesity becoming an epidemic?
Obesity is already an epidemic, and it's out of control. Globally, there are more than one billion overweight adults, at least 300 million of them are obese. As for the United States, and reported by the CDC (Centers for Disease Control), obesity rose 33% in the last decade with an *astounding 65%* of our population now considered obese. 65%?! Quite frankly, one only has to look around to see that number is probably closer to 85-90%. (COVID has made this far worse.) Either or, it's hard to fathom. If this trend continues, experts say 95% of all Americans will be obese by the year 2040. Needless to say, adults need do whatever it takes to break this cycle for themselves and their children. It's not just the visual aspect of being overweight that's so terribly distressing, more so, the many illnesses and diseases that are caused by eating poorly.

According to the National Center of Health Statistics:
A breakdown of approximately 127 million adults are overweight, 60 million are obese, and 9 million are morbidly obese. Obesity in children has caused an epidemic of diabetes. Estimated annual U.S. healthcare costs due to obesity are over $117 billion, $10 billion more than all forms of cancer. Obesity is now the second leading cause of preventable death, surpassed only by smoking. Each year an estimated 300,000 Americans die from disease caused by being overweight. As of 2000, there were 400,000 obesity-related deaths. It's now shy just 15,000 of becoming the #1 preventable death! **UPDATE**: As of 2020, a recent study shows that 42.4% of people living in the U.S. are obese. I simply must ask: *How did it ever come to this?* Well, I think we all know the answer by now.

NEWS FLASH: Our government is suddenly claiming the death toll from obesity is only 112,000 not 400,000. *Why the drastic change?* This is due to the relentless pressure by the lobbyists for the food industry. Shockingly, this same report is also claiming, and I quote, "People who are modestly overweight, but not obese, have a lower risk of death than people of normal weight." *Reeeeally?* Where are the studies to support these highly questionable claims? This is insane. Does no one question their motives? This retraction, and self-serving health claim, are both based entirely on the food industry trying to make sure we keep eating their poisoned food. This will ensure we stay fat, addicted, and riddled with disease. This action proves, yet again, it is about greed and profits—and all at the consumer's expense. Not to mention, this kind of commentary coming from our own damn government will give those who are overweight, a license to keep on eating, without guilt, care, or concern.

I can't believe they could be so far off. It makes me seriously question their intentions. So how do food companies get us addicted?
Getting the consumer addicted to their products can be easily accomplished, either by adding sugar on the front end, using ingredients that have naturally occurring sugar, or by using high GI carbs that *turn into* sugar once consumed. To further confuse the consumer, they cleverly hide all kinds of sugar in their products under many different names, names that most people will not recognize as sugar. If that isn't enough, food manufacturers also add certain chemicals that can cause addiction. It's very simple. These companies only make money if you continue to buy their products. Hence, they will do whatever it takes to keep you coming back for more, regardless of how this food affects your health. Again, it's all about profits. Period. *And then our government wonders why we are all so fat—and getting sicker by the minute?*

Didn't someone file a "fat suit?"
Yes, back in July 2002, a gentleman filed a major lawsuit against the fast food industry, claiming fast food is addictive, which, subsequently, led to his two heart attacks. The suit charged the biggest names in the industry for basically not informing him, the public, that their food was inordinately unhealthy and addictive. Though I believe such companies should offer healthier food choices, it's up to us as individuals to know what we're eating. Although we are forever enticed through TV ads, billboards, $1 specials, playgrounds, toys, even ATMs for stress-free purchase, no one forced this man to eat this food. On the other hand, this type of food is highly addictive and always in our face. These companies spend billions of dollars on seductive ad campaigns, targeting primarily the younger generation. Their marketing approach is precise: "Get 'em hooked while they're young!" Therefore, the fast food industry should be held liable to a certain degree. Better yet, maybe this lawsuit will bring about some positive changes to this industry. In the meantime, think for yourself and make better food choices. Maintaining your serotonin will control your cravings for junk food.

UPDATE: Since this lawsuit was filed, some changes have been made in the fast food industry. Burger King is offering a veggie burger. I'd be terribly concerned what's in it. Several other chains are offering salads, fruit plates, egg white muffin, and bottled water. Love the water, however, the salads are loaded with dried fruit, bread crumbs, etc. Egg white muffin is equally not healthy. Sadly, these offerings are based on the low fat myth.

If you still believe eating fast food is without health risks, I insist you watch the highly acclaimed documentary "SUPER SIZE ME" by filmmaker Morgan Spurlock. This man risked his very life to show the public just how toxic fast food is. Beyond how terribly sick this food made him, you'll see how it equally affected him mentally and emotionally. Happy one minute. Depressed the next. This is directly related to insulin being spiked by the high GI carbs, which then increases the production of serotonin. Hence, being called comfort food. Unfortunately, the serotonin will soon plummet. Followed by craving more of the same. The same old, unhealthy cycle.

Any concerns with the healthier options offered by fast food restaurants?
Even though they're offering pretended healthier options, this food still contains damaged fats and carcinogens, along with plenty of hidden sugars and addictive chemicals. After all, how else will these restaurants keep you coming back for more? Once again, it is all about profits. You really should AVOID fast food at all cost. If there is no other option (which there always will be), I suggest the salads, minus the croutons. For those who want something other than a salad, I suggest either a chicken breast or a burger wrapped in lettuce, both without the bun. Avoid coffee, sodas, and juice. Drink water. Avoid salad dressings and condiments, as they're high in sugar and chemicals. Lemon, olive oil, and vinegar make a wonderful dressing. As for their fruit plates, please avoid. I sincerely hope it isn't necessary to say that you should not be eating the hash browns, muffins, pancakes, bagels, onion rings, french fries, french toast, breakfast burritos, McNuggets, tacos, taco salads, fried chicken, egg rolls, rice bowls, cookies, frozen parfaits, McFlurries, milk shakes, or deep-fried cherry pies?

In closing this chapter, I want to applaud the many schools across the country for having the courage to take a stand against childhood obesity. These school systems are removing soda and candy machines, eliminating processed and refined food, and replacing them with freshly prepared real food. In a very short time, the teachers are already noticing a remarkable difference in the students' energy level, attention span, and overall attitude. Little do they know, but this is only the beginning. Parents and teachers alike would be astonished to see just how quickly their kids would slim down and no longer suffer from outbursts of rage, ADD/ADHD, mood swings, etc., once they're off this addictive, deadly, junk food. Can you possibly imagine how many pharmaceutical drugs would no longer be needed to treat the many professed "diseases" kids, teens, and adults are suffering from due to this food? People would be astonished at how healthy they could get and how great they could feel.

Finally, success in fat loss is far more than just a number on a scale. It's about achieving excellent health of both body and mind, as well as truly liking yourself, inside and out. I want you to be *modestly* confident in all that you are. I want you to love and respect yourself.

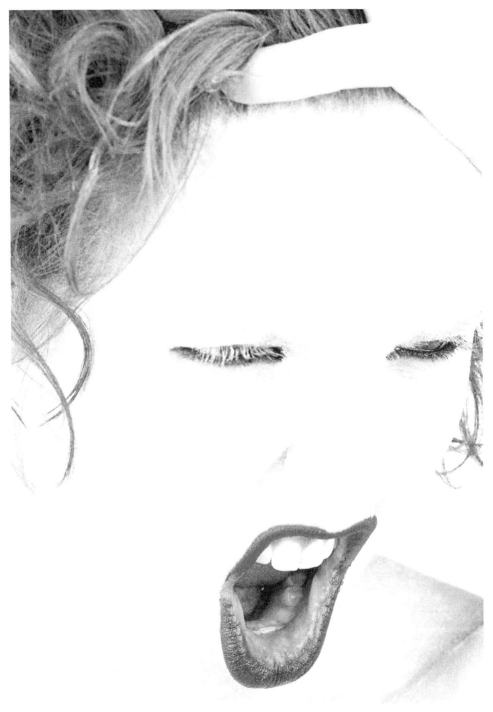

16

FAT CELLS GETTIN' FATTER

You mentioned fat cells. *You said we have how many?*
An adult who is at normal weight has approximately 20–27 billion fat cells. An adult who is overweight can have fat cells that range in numbers from 75 billion to over 300 billion. One amazing fact is that fat cells do not multiply after puberty, i.e., as your body stores more fat, the actual number of fat cells remains the same. Each fat cell, instead, gets bigger. Fat cells also increase far more rapidly in obese children than in thin children. The amount of fat someone has, is a reflection of both the number and the size of their fat cells. And, I'm sorry to say, but due to various factors, women have more.

Billions? Oooh, no! Can I ever get rid of them?
Not exactly. We all know, especially women, just how damn easy it is to fill up our fat cells. Fat cells can shrink, but they don't ever just disappear. Liposuction can remove some of your fat cells, but unless you're able to control your cravings, you will never maintain the fat loss. You will eventually, as with all your diets in the past, succumb to the cravings and put the weight back on, plus some. You must also be willing to make other necessary changes. Your new, healthy lifestyle must include not only healthy food and habits, but it must also include regular exercise. If not, the fat cells will again grow in number and continue to enlarge.

Do overweight people have a harder time shrinking their fat cells?
Overweight people have an extra hard time losing excess body fat, because not only do they have more fat cells (about three times as many), their fat cells are also now about a third bigger than those at their normal weight. So, yes, those people who are overweight have more fat cells, which can be more difficult to shrink.

It seems absolutely hopeless! What can I do?
The more fat cells a person has, the harder it will be to lose weight. That's not to say that you can't lose it, with effort and long-term commitment. This is why you need to start making a serious effort <u>today</u> to lose the excess body fat. You must also teach your children good, healthy eating and lifestyle habits starting today. They might not like it at first, but they will, without a doubt, thank you later.

What are fat cells used for?
Fat cells are used by the body to store excess calories. Calories are energy, used by the body for future use. The energy that your body uses today, may be coming from a meal you ate weeks, or even several months, prior. Just remember, the excess calories that

your body does not utilize for energy is promoted to fat storage. All the more reason you need to build lean muscle, as muscle is a metabolically active tissue, far more active than fat and, as such, it requires a precise number of calories daily to maintain itself. More muscle = *more calories burned*.

Okay, but why do I feel fat from my ankles up after a high-carb meal?
Some of the bloating comes from those carbs triggering your insulin, which then leads to a higher level of sodium. In addition, a high-carb meal, of course, also opens your fat cells, causing them to store new fat. Ironically, this reminds me of my own struggles from many years ago. Please allow me to share:

Childhood memories...

I was one of 7 children, raised in the Midwest with pretty typical eating habits: Finish what's on your plate, eat three square meals, with my stepmother always freshly preparing anything from ham, pot roast, pork chops, meatloaf, chicken, etc. These dishes were accompanied by a variety of veggies, potatoes, salads, and desserts. There was also my father's Saturday morning breakfast of eggs, bacon, and cinnamon toast and the Friday evening yippee-the-parents-are-going-out-quick-fix-meals, everything from hot dogs, sizzle steaks, fish sticks, Sloppy Joe's, tater tots, mac' and cheese, pot pies, french fries, and an abundance of s'mores. In and around all of the traditional food, we still managed to eat copious amounts of sugar-coated cereal, pancakes, Pop-tarts, Wonder Bread sandwiches, potato chips, Snowballs, Ding-Dongs, and Twinkies. I'll never forget how my younger brother Tommy and I would race our bikes down to the lake front store nearly every day, eager to spend our weekly allowance. We'd take our tiny, but overflowing brown paper bags filled with nickel candy, washing each sweet delight down with delicious sugar-laden ice cold pops and then proceed to look for trouble.

Lucky for me, I was a tomboy, never sitting still. I'm sure I burned up the excessive overload of sugar by chasing the boys, then running *from* the boys, playing red-rover, duck-duck-goose, hide-and-seek, kick-the-can, and racing my brother's motorcycles. Then there was tag football, shootin' hoops, horseback riding, water skiing, swimming, and the many athletic sports I played through school. As kids we never stopped. Like cattle, my stepmother would literally have to ring a huge bell to get us to come home.

Later on, though, as a young woman, I came to believe I wasn't meant to eat. I came to this startling conclusion because I had long given up the candy and the many other things we were told were unhealthy. (Even way back then, it was all about low fat.) But I still began to gain weight. I had always been so athletic and lean, but things seemed to be changing. I was not happy. All I'd have was a toasted bagel with some orange juice and only moments later, I felt like a blow fish. I felt so fat, but why? I had eaten so little, yet my pants were suddenly tight! I felt bloated! Aggravated. Bitchy. Tired. *Why, though?* I couldn't understand *how* I could feel so fat and moody. After all, I only had a bagel and a lousy glass of fruit juice. I mean, come on, a bagel had NO fat! The juice was from fruit, which was all-natural. Again, no fat. So how could I be gaining weight? To make matters worse, I was hungry all the time, never felt satiated, and the only food I craved was more of the same. Ahhh, I was miserable and awfully frustrated.

That sounds just like me!
I felt it was important to share the above story, as I'm sure there are many adults, teens, and even children, who can relate to this exact scenario. The truth of the matter is, I was eating the "recommended diet" provided by the AMA and the FDA. Both my bagel and juice fell perfectly within their guidelines of low fat dieting. They were indeed low fat, but, unfortunately, extremely high in sugar and high GI carbs. Based on what you've just learned here, you now know precisely why my body and mind reacted the way they did. Moreover, why their recommended low fat dieting did not work. In fact, low fat dieting is one of the biggest direct contributors to our current rate of obesity.

Obviously, this was long before I ever began my research. But, as you can see, even four decades ago, I was learning to listen to my body. By doing so, I began to understand, on my own, what food my body thrived on. I discovered that when I ate fruit, more so, when I drank fruit juice, I could actually feel the sugar rush through my system. It made me feel terribly hyped. Caffeine, whether it came from sodas or coffee, also made me feel far too anxious, followed by mood swings and a severe drop in energy. Cereal, chips, and bagels were all very comforting, but I never felt full, at least for very long. I also felt bloated after eating that food. Eventually, I began to avoid them and instead leaned toward cheese, eggs, chicken, and...diet sodas. Yes, diet sodas. I was still learning. I hate to think of all the aspartame I've consumed.

The junk food I ate as a child is not terribly different from what the kids eat today, but we always had a base of healthy food, followed by the less than desirable treats. The biggest differences: We ate mostly home-cooked meals, rarely if ever eating fast food, and we were always physically active. Not only have schools stopped scheduling Physical Education (which I find astounding), but the kids don't motivate themselves to play. Parents need to make them turn off the TV, computer, video games, and get their not-so little butts moving. Sedentary lifestyles are a major contributor to obesity in children, teens, and adults. This is precisely why we're suddenly seeing so many new cases of diabetes. In addition to balancing your serotonin, this is a perfect example of where a dramatic change in lifestyle is desperately needed.

Personal reflection: As I grocery shopped today, I was truly shocked by how many obese people I saw. Nearly every single person was at least 60-80 pounds overweight and with nothing, but unhealthy food in their grocery carts. The harsh reality is, most don't give a damn about what their food will do to them. They eat solely for selfish pleasure. No regard to their health, that is, not until D-I-S-E-A-S-E comes knocking.

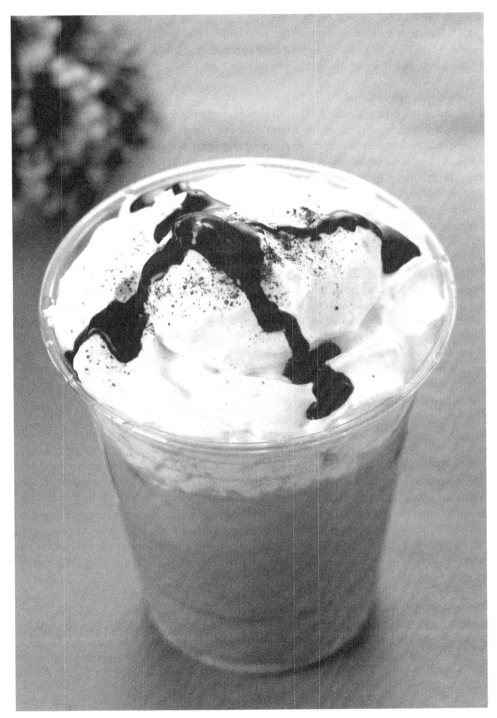

17

ALL STIMULANTS BECOME DEPRESSANTS
"Got coffee?"

My latte will do what?
All stimulants become depressants, be it your latte, wine, high GI carbs, sugar, various drugs, beer, and much more. This happens, because all stimulants first elevate serotonin, but within an hour or two, *those serotonin levels will most certainly drop*. The brain will then begin to struggle. It will start to push you toward more of the same junk food/drink that elevated your serotonin to begin with, which leads to mood swings, rage, depression, anxiety, panic attacks, and so on. Not to mention, you'll also be storing more body fat.

This pattern is precisely why millions of people worldwide are depressed, anxious, and suffering with panic attacks. They call it "MENTAL ILLNESS." No, for the most part, it is simply low levels of serotonin due to the terribly unhealthy lifestyle habits most people take part in. Who doesn't start their day with Starbucks? Sadly, millions worldwide do.

How does that happen?
Remember, serotonin, among many things, governs our mental/emotional health. It is the master communicator of all brain chemicals. For the brain and body to function at its best, it must be maintained. I plead with you to please learn all the things that will deplete your serotonin, that is, if you want to live free of depression, anxiety, mood swings, rage, etc.

Unfortunately, most people start their day with caffeine and end it with wine. *This is a serious addictive pattern.* Nearly every woman that seeks my help, starts her day with 2-3 cups of coffee and ends it with 1-2 glasses of wine. And, they're on antidepressant(s), or they wish they were. They're anxious, overweight, exhausted, and with high trigs/low HDL.

Sounds like me! No wonder I feel so awful!
Stimulants deplete serotonin, causing depression, anxiety, insomnia, agitation, and continued carb cravings. However, they also cause the body to produce a harmful form of cholesterol which can lead to heart disease, high blood pressure, stroke, diabetes, Alzheimer's etc. Bottom line: You can't use stimulants, no matter the form they come in, if you want to achieve a healthy body and mind. It requires commitment, consistency, and knowing long-term weight loss is about a *healthy lifestyle,* not a quick fix with stimulants.

Oprah and Prince Harry recently produced a docu series, "The Me You Can't See." It was about the alarming statistics on so-called mental illness around the world, especially since COVID. I would agree more people are suffering, but here's why: Stress is one of the key things that will deplete serotonin. When we're stressed, our serotonin levels plummet. We then start to consume the food/drink that will elevate this brain chemical. I'm quite sure caffeine and wine sales skyrocketed since COVID. However, this is exactly why so many people are suffering with mental health issues due to this pattern. This is also why so many people gained weight during the pandemic. Look at the cycle. It is science based. But drugs are not the answer.

I'm not saying that some people might truly have mental health issues, but more often than not, depression and anxiety can be alleviated by simply changing one's nutrition, using the right form and dose of magnesium, getting them off all stimulants, and, of course, using the 5 to safely, and effectively, elevate their serotonin. What I found fascinating is that with all the many mental health experts featured in that doc-series, no one ever mentioned how our nutrition, stimulants, alcohol, etc., play a critical role in our mental/emotional health. *How can that be?* No one?

SIMPLE FACT:
Eat crap. Feel like crap, *physically and mentally.*

I have personally weaned dozens of clients off antidepressants, while alleviating their depression and anxiety. I weaned one woman off two antidepressants and an anxiety med, along with her junk carbs, caffeine, and wine in just two months. She told me she had never felt this good before. Her husband said he felt like he went through a divorce, got a new wife, and all without the expense of a divorce. In all modesty, I do this nearly every month with the people who seek my help. If you know nutrition, and you know how to implement the science that my research is based, it is effortless.

Why don't you recommend stimulants for fat loss?
Products that use stimulants to speed up your metabolism are harmful and unhealthy. (This includes the Brazilian diet pills. Among other ingredients, the morning dose contains speed. The evening dose contains Prozac and Valium. Stay clear of these, and other appetite suppressants such as Hoodia.) Stimulants put excessive stress on your adrenal glands and heart. For those millions of people who are told they need to be on lifelong thyroid medication, the excessive stress brought on by stimulants is most often a contributing factor. Although you may lose pounds according to the scale, most often it's from lean muscle mass and water, <u>not</u> fat. Moreover, once you go off these stimulant-based diet products and begin to eat normally, you'll most likely gain all the weight back, plus some. This relates directly to the old "lose 10/gain back 20" scenario. With each new attempt to diet, it will be even harder to lose the fat. What you've done instead is risk your health, drastically reduce your lean muscle mass, change your total body composition, thereby, *increasing* your fat stores. While it may seem you're losing fat quicker with stimulants, it's a false and unhealthy fix, not a lifelong solution. Furthermore, you have not learned "how or why" the body stores fat, or <u>why</u> you crave high GI carbs/sugar.

Stims also trigger insulin, directly or indirectly, as they trigger cortisol and promote the breakdown of glycogen. The breakdown of glycogen causes the liver to release glucose into the bloodstream. (Glucose is the most potent stimulant of insulin release.) This triggers the pancreas to secret excess insulin, which leads to a sharp blood sugar drop (hypoglycemia). Once insulin is spiked, it encourages the storage of body fat. Stims also increase weight gain due to salt and water retention.

Different type of stimulants would include?
Stimulant sources are endless and vary from prescription/nonprescription drugs, OTC (Over the Counter) meds, to ephedra, caffeine, sugar, chocolate, high GI carbs, nicotine, sexual enhancing herbs, alcohol, soda, chocolate milk, cocoa, to your frappuccino, etc.

How do you feel about phentermine? My doctor offers it to me.
In addition to the many health concerns just mentioned, I would never suggest such drugs, as phentermine. This is not the way you want to lose weight. It is unhealthy and short-lived.

Personally, I am overly sensitive to stimulants. I also hate that feeling of being amped, on edge, or unable to sleep. Thus, I do whatever it takes to avoid them. That would include ephedrine, caffeine, yohimbe, guarana, etc. Ironically, my first supplier of raw ingredients feverishly tried to convince me that, because I refused to use ephedra (or any other stimulant), I was "missing the boat and failing to realize the *real needs* in the weight loss market." When I explained my research, he was condescending, claiming I was being foolish and making a huge mistake as a product developer. He then accused me of trying to change the world. I humbly replied, "Yes, I suppose I am."

His next attempt to force my hand was to remind me that Walmart's best-seller was Metabolife, an ephedra-based weight loss product. Again, I told him I didn't care. More importantly, I'd be nothing more than a pathetic hypocrite if I used it, as it was against everything I knew to be healthy, for weight loss or otherwise. I explained to him that while people may lose weight with stims, it was unhealthy, and they would more than likely gain all the weight back after they went off those products, as they had not learned why they crave all those insulin-producing carbs. His quick reply was, "Perfect. You just sell them another product!"

Sorry. This approach is not at all who I am, or how I work. I'm not some self-righteous woman either, but it's unfortunately terribly common in our industry. All one has to do is read the ingredients (and deceptive claims) on any given product, to realize that far too many companies do not give a damn about their customers, rather, it's only about profit margins. This is also a perfect example of standing up for what you believe in, learning to think for yourself, and never letting yourself be manipulated by guilt or money.

To learn even more about how nutrition and our mental health are connected, please read my next chapter.

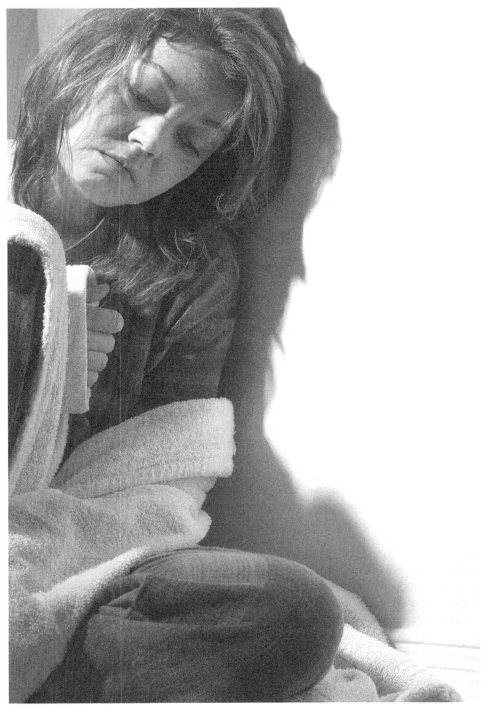

18

DIRECT LINK BETWEEN
MENTAL HEALTH & OUR NUTRITION
You are what you eat; physically & mentally

How exactly does our diet affect our mental health?
No matter the underlying trigger(s), depression is due to the depletion of serotonin, the major neurotransmitter among all brain chemicals. Each year depression strikes over an astounding 17 million adults, teens, and children in the U.S. Over 12 million diagnosed are women. Since COVID, these numbers are far worse. They are at alarming, epidemic proportions. Remember, serotonin is depleted by many things. In addition to stress, a few primary contributing factors are the over-consumption of processed/refined carbs, sodas, caffeine, nicotine, high GI carbs, sugar, HFCS and artificial sweeteners. Regrettably, Americans consume these in excessive amounts.

Are you saying my coffee and food choices can cause depression?
Yes. Who doesn't start their day with a couple cups of coffee with some decadent, candy-bar-in-a-bottle-creamer, with pasta for lunch, followed by wine with dinner? I see this same unhealthy pattern with nearly every single client that I work. It is, alarmingly, an epidemic of endless addictions that will lead to so-called "mental illness." Yet it is nothing more than coming to understand all the things that you're consuming on a daily basis, are constantly depleting your serotonin levels.

How does this happen?
To reiterate, the caffeine (and junk carbs) will elevate your serotonin, but then drop it pretty quickly. In addition to triggering your insulin (and putting your body into fat storage mode), your brain will then struggle until you give into another source that will, once again, elevate your serotonin levels, hence, the pasta (or sub) midday, with wine, beer or vodka at dinner. Yet then everyone wonders why they're so damn anxious all the time, depressed, on meds, can't sleep, pants are tight, miserable, and feel and look much older than they should. It is a vicious cycle of low serotonin, cravings, caffeine, alcohol, sugar, weight gain, mood swings, anxiety, depression, repeat, repeat, repeat. My absolute amazement comes from the fact that no one, and I mean, NO ONE, is talking about the direct link between mental health—and our nutrition. It frustrates me to no end, because millions are suffering.

I'm shocked by this, because my psychiatrist has never spoken to me about how my coffee and/or wine could be the root of my depression and endless anxiety.
I find it very upsetting, because, once again, no one in the medical industry ever questions the direct link between depression and our nutrition. Never have I heard anyone

say that when they spoke to their doctor about their depression, that doctor ever asked, inquired, and/or expressed concern about their "nutrition." It simply does not happen. It's far easier, not to mention financially more rewarding, to prescribe yet another drug. In lieu of our doctors, AMA and FDA promoting wellness and preventive methods of treatment and educating people about how to eat a healthy, nutritious diet, combined with efficacious herbal supplementation to *naturally* alleviate depression and anxiety, they'd rather prescribe DRUGS, be it Prozac, Zoloft, Xanax, or another harmful drug.

It's truly shocking how the U.S. pharmaceutical industry has been glorifying their many antidepressant drugs. For example, a certain TV commercial: *"Do you have a special event coming up? A family affair? A celebration? Call your doctor today to see if you're eligible for Prozac Weekly!"* This advertisement was terribly alarming. It seductively played more like a beer commercial. More disturbing yet is that they found it acceptable to treat depression, to offer happiness, for only a week at a time.

In lieu of the medical community making the necessary effort to find out the underlying causes of depression, anxiety, panic attacks, etc, they'd rather sell a drug to *mask* the symptoms. Remember, these pharmaceutical drugs are just that, D-R-U-G-S, all of which will lead to serious side effects. People need to realize they can help take control of their mental health by supporting healthy levels of serotonin, *naturally*. If you question the deadly side effects of these drugs, drugs that Big Pharma actually manipulated their clinical findings, I urge you to read *The Shooting Drugs, Prozac Exposed* by Donna Smart. It documents hundreds of terrifying cases of those who went on psychotic rampages brutally murdering their families, strangers, classmates, then committing suicide, *all while on antidepressants.* (Columbine is merely one example.) It also documents the depth to which the drug companies will go to protect the future sales of their deadly drugs, i.e., bribery, threats, falsifying records, etc. You must read this book before taking any antidepressant.

If this discussion isn't enough to concern you, I once met a psychiatrist in passing. I was sincerely intrigued by his work. But when I questioned if he ever discussed how his patients' diets played a critical role in their mental health, he looked at me with a cold blank stare and said, *"Why* would I do that? Their diet has <u>nothing</u> to do with their depression!" *Excuse me?* This doctor wasn't just a family practitioner from whom you might expect such a limited understanding. He was a licensed and practicing psychiatrist. Hell, the minute I think I can eat or drink something that is less than my usual healthy choices, my anxiety will kick in. *You are what you eat.* Never forget that. It is not mental illness.

FACT: Less than 2% of all doctors are trained in nutrition. Those teachings are based on the low fat myth, and the class is often only one damn week. Most medical students don't even opt for that brief course. I find this astounding, considering most diseases are nutritionally based. How can this be considered acceptable? Again, I urge you to educate yourself. Research. Commit to a healthier lifestyle starting today. Seek out a health expert who will treat the depression, <u>minus</u> drugs. Whatever choice you make, weigh the benefits and the many risks. Never forgetting, we're not meant to be "happy" every moment of our lives. As human beings, we will experience countless emotions.

Alarming statistic: The fastest-growing market for antidepressants is preschool children. To imagine these children being drugged, at an age when their young minds are developing most, is horrendous. *Why is this being allowed?* The drug companies will stop at nothing. Do not be fooled by their self-serving diagnosis. Research on your own. Get a second, even third opinion. Use a PDR (Prescription Drug Reference) to substantiate side effects, which will be numerous and life-threatening. No disrespect intended, but I cannot believe parents would allow this without questioning such a harmful prescription. (This also pertains to the drugs doctors are prescribing for ADD/ADHD, etc.)

So, before you, and especially your children, start taking these drugs, take a closer look at what you/yours are eating and drinking. Based on what you've learned, thus far, you now know that diet plays a CRITICAL role in your mental and emotional health. Therefore, take a fresh look at all the food and beverages (as well as nicotine and alcohol) you and your family consume on any given day. Then make the much-needed changes. More than likely, it will not be easy weaning off the highly processed junk food, as your brain will continue to tempt you with the carbs that it knows has always triggered the production of serotonin. However, 5-HTP will absolutely help people control these endless cravings.

I've noticed my mother is also depressed. What can I do for her?
Due to age, often failing health, and the far too many meds that most seniors are on, combined with a diet that is terribly high in sugar, caffeine, alcohol, etc., their mental health is often dramatically affected. Statistics prove one of the biggest health concerns with seniors is depression. From my own personal experience, I've been blessed throughout my life to befriend many amazing elderly people. Whether I met them as neighbors, at my gym, or simply by going to visit local retirement or nursing homes, I've always had an incredible attraction to those much older than myself. There is such an honesty there, no pretense, no games, no ulterior motives, just pure, raw thoughts and emotions shared between two human beings. Through these friendships, though, I've witnessed the kinds of meals they eat, either those they prepared themselves or were served in the homes. From morning till night, they also eagerly consume an endless array of sugar and caffeine, from iced teas and coffee, sodas, juice, candy, etc. Add to that the often questionable meals they eat and the far too many senseless pharma drugs they take, which, of course, also deplete serotonin, and well, I'm sure the next time you, their loving and devoted child go to visit them, you'll know exactly *why* they're so depressed.

But what can I do?
Please take what you've learned here and help them. Be there for them. Spend time with them. If they live in a home, do not assume these homes have your parents' best interest at heart. You need to be their advocate. Visit them often. Make sure they're eating healthy. Don't let their doctor overload them with senseless drugs. Take them for walks. Have lunch

with them. Read to them. Stimulate their minds and emotions. Be part of their life. Don't let them feel forgotten. Though you may not be able to care for them full time, at least do whatever it takes to make sure the time they do have left is lived with a clear and emotionally fulfilled mind. The time you spend with them, and with the many other residents who will literally beg you to get them out of there, will surely make you cry or, at the very least, make you wish you could do more for them. I also sincerely hope it will further inspire you to live a much healthier life. Being able to maintain healthy levels of serotonin with the 5 can be extremely beneficial, and more importantly, *without* side effects. In addition to helping control cravings, the 5 can also enhance mood, sleep patterns, energy, etc. This supplement can indeed offer you, and your aging parents, many positive health benefits.

Caffeine, the #1 socially accepted, legalized D-R-U-G.

My mother is on way too many drugs. She also has 3 or 4 cups of coffee before noon, plus, several iced teas. By the way, isn't caffeine a drug?
Yes, all the more reason to be concerned. Caffeine is the #1 socially accepted, legalized drug. Caffeine also happens to be highly addictive. Caffeine, along with the sweet taste of added sugar, is the reason why sodas are consumed by our youth (and adults, too) at a startling rate of 54 gallons per person, per year. This doesn't include the caffeine you can get from your local coffee café. I most certainly respect Starbucks business savvy, but people seem to forget that caffeine is a <u>drug,</u> and it plays a major role in their inability to lose excess body fat, stabilize their mood, improve cholesterol panels, etc.

Starbucks currently has 32,938 locations worldwide, with $24 BILLION in sales. Statistics show that roughly 60 million people visit Starbucks every week, going on an average of 18 times per month. (Since COVID, I'm quite sure that's doubled.) Besides the excessive amount of caffeine, at a <u>minimum</u> of $7, plus a $2 tip, this caffeine habit alone adds up to no less than $162 per month, $1,944 per year. And, unless you're wearing blinders, how can anyone possibly resist their wickedly decadent pastries that scream to be eaten. Sweets were never my weakness, but when they're in your face like that teasing you, *tempting you,* well, no wonder most people succumb to this manipulative sugar-tease. (Thankfully, I remain in control, because my serotonin is balanced.)

Nevertheless, 18 times a month you enjoy a latte (plain, nonfat, large latte = 30g carbs/sugar), with maybe a sesame bagel (440 calories, 630mg sodium, 92g carbs/sugar), or maybe a chocolate cream cheese muffin (450 calories, 420mg sodium, 53g carbs/sugar). Add this to your other not-so-healthy daily habits. Now can you start to see why so many people are stressed out, on edge, depressed, suffering from insomnia, alarming cholesterol panels, sexually unavailable, and quickly gaining weight?

But I enjoy a cup of coffee with my friends. What should I do?
I'm not saying you can't enjoy a cup of coffee, just please consider drinking *water processed decaf* coffee, better yet, caffeine free herbal tea. You also need to be aware of all

the sugar in those flavored syrup blends, and the milk, nonfat or otherwise. Do not add sugar or artificial sweeteners.

MARKETING PLOY: Starbucks, like many others, are very clever with their products and how they market them to the trusting consumer. On the front of Starbucks Thai-Style Peanut Chicken Wrap, with grapes, they proudly boast 450 calories, 11g protein, and 4g fiber. But hold up. Don't fall for that self-serving marketing hype. Read the Nutrition Facts and Ingredient Panels. What about the 47g of carbs, 20g of which are sugar? Let's not forget the EDTA, soybean oil, cornstarch, maltodextrin, etc., that's in this proclaimed healthy food. The chemicals alone are alarming, but, because all carbs, minus the fiber, equal sugar, that would be 43g of sugar. Please read all labels.

Why don't you use nonfat milk?
I'm glad you asked this, because I hear so many people ordering their lattes and frappuccinos and it's always with nonfat milk. Unfortunately, the fear of dietary fat still runs rampant. You're actually better off using milk *with* the fat, hence, my heavy whipping cream, as the fat actually helps lower the blood sugar response from the sugar naturally found in milk. Yes, you heard me right. The fat is a good thing. Our bodies need fat for many reasons. The fat helps lower the glycemic response. Skim, 2%, 1%, low-fat, or nonfat milk still contain plenty of lactose (milk sugar), but without any fat, this milk will affect blood sugar levels much more dramatically.

You're right, it makes perfect sense. But what are your concerns with soy?
Soy and its many food products were touted as the best thing out there, but studies are now showing otherwise. Soy food products made from soy protein powders, soy protein isolates, textured soy proteins, as well as soy milk, have been shown to contain both natural and added chemicals. These chemicals are proving to be harmful to the body. For starters, non-fermented soy products contain phytic acid, which contains anti-nutritive properties. Phytic acid binds with certain nutrients, including iron, to inhibit their absorption.

"Got milk?" GAIN WEIGHT.

And your concerns with cow's milk are?
First of all, cow's milk is intended for baby calves. There are numerous studies that clearly demonstrate just how unhealthy cow's milk is for humans. All the while, the NDC (National Dairy Council) spends millions of dollars on clever ad campaigns. "Got milk?" is the most successful ad by far. However, I find one of their recent ads, an ad that shows men eagerly scrambling to buy as much milk as possible, because they're claiming milk "may" help reduce symptoms of PMS, is misinformed—and insulting to women.

I'm ecstatic to report that their latest campaign, a campaign that has cost over $200 million, has prompted lawsuits against the biggest names, i.e., Dannon, Kraft, General Mills, etc. The ad claims, "Drinking 24 oz. of milk per day may help people lose weight, particularly belly fat." *Reeeeally?* "Got studies?" Oh, of course they do, but guess who funded the studies? The NDC. Hence, their deceptive claims. Michael Zemel, professor of nutrition/medicine at the University of TN, received $1.7 million in research grants since 1998 to secure statistics that would support their campaign. Obviously he was unsuccessful. Thus, the lawsuits. Milk will not help people lose weight. And because it's a liquid carb—and people most often only drink fat free milk—it will actually *encourage* weight gain. *Can you say moo?* (BTW: Where is the FDA, the FTC? Hmmm? Why have they allowed these ads to run so long without holding the NDC accountable for their fraudulent claims? Yet another example of the disreputable, illegal, and harmful relationship between big business and our government.)

Furthermore, cow's milk contains many harmful components. Proteins in cow's milk are different from human milk proteins. It causes problems with digestion, impaired absorption of other nutrients, intolerance, and autoimmune reactions. Few of the proteins meant for a calf are found naturally in human mother's milk, and none are found in any natural adult human food. In addition, cow hormones are not meant for humans. Over time, cows have been selectively bred to create high levels of these exact hormones, those that help cows to grow the fastest and produce the greatest amount of milk. There is also a high concentration of pesticides and pollutants in cow's milk. The high amount of drugs now given to cows makes this all the more serious.

I thought milk was required for building strong bones?
This is precisely what the NDC has perpetuated for decades. It is not factual. The high protein content of milk actually causes a net loss of calcium in the body. Studies that were even paid for by the NDC have shown that the excessive protein in milk lowers blood calcium levels, causing the body to actually draw on calcium from the bones. The advertising propaganda put forth by the NDC with regard to drinking milk to prevent osteoporosis is inaccurate. Milk can actually encourage this medical condition. I realize most of you will not believe this, so I urge you to research this further on your own. The studies are clear.

Damn! More deceit, more frustration! What do you suggest?
Be aware of the health risks, but then make the best choices possible. Personally, I eat plenty of non-starchy vegetables and assorted fresh cheeses, organic whenever possible. Again, using unsweetened almond milk with my tea. Also, please don't forget that dairy cows are forced to endure such awful lives, as well as being slaughtered as soon as they are no longer able to produce milk. Their innocent lives are filled with abuse, and then cut terribly short. Lastly, by consuming cow's milk, even cheese, we inadvertently support the veal industry. I certainly want no more part of that torture. So please, try to limit your products from cows, as I sincerely try to do.

What if I make my coffee at home and use a flavored coffee creamer?
Anything that tastes that sweet cannot possibly be good. There are many varieties of these richly delicious creamers, and not one is a healthy choice. *Why?* Because they're loaded

with sugar. Read the nutrition and ingredient panels. The first ingredient: water. The second: sugar or corn syrup solids. The serving size is 1 tbsp. It equals 5g of sugar. If that isn't enough, is anyone really going to use just one little tbsp? I think not.

Once again, it is about choices and picking your occasional treat. But stop and ask yourself: Considering these creamers are nothing more than sugar water, then added to caffeine, both of which will spike your insulin, deplete your serotonin, put your body into a fat-storing mode for hours, cause bloating and mood swings, and even further perpetuate carb cravings and fat gain, why, then, would you want to use them?

Confession: Long before Starbucks, I bought those sinfully delicious creamers to top off my equally decadent flavored decaf coffee to enjoy at home. *Ooooh, both were so good!* I knew the creamers were pretty much pure sugar, but I figured, because it was my one and only treat, I was entitled. *Wasn't I?* I mean, come on, how bad could they be? Well, I can assure you I don't feel this way any longer. Ironically, even after I became fully aware of the dangers of the ingredients, both in the creamers and soothing cup of Joe, my brain kept quietly, but continually forcing me toward that sweet delight. It wasn't until I started developing my 5-based supps that I finally got rid of the craving for this syrupy drink. And while I could, like many others, simply keep on enjoying this warm sugar concoction, even though the craving was long gone, I could no longer ignore the numerous health risks associated with sugar, corn syrup, etc. Eliminating them from my diet is simply one more way to help keep my body as lean as possible, my moods stable, and my energy constant.

Point taken. I'll leave the creamer out. Should I stop drinking coffee altogether?

In a perfect world, yes. At the same time, I would never tell you or anyone else what to do. Nonetheless, I would hope that you'd consider drinking *water processed* decaf. My only intention is to educate you. It is then your decision, as to what you will do with this information. This brings me to an interesting observation: I'm probably like a lot of women who don't really care about the caffeine. It's more the habit, the tradition of making coffee first thing in the morning. The grinding of fresh coffee beans. The intoxicating aroma as it permeates the house. Maybe meeting the girls out to socialize and then taking that first glorious sip. Ahhhh, it triggers such a wonderful sensation! Well, here's the good news: You can still enjoy all of that without the health risks associated with caffeine.

Furthermore, ladies, for those who have men in their life who think they need caffeine to start their day, I suggest you start weaning them off it with decaf. Day by day cut it back, until it is only pure decaf. Most will never miss it. Trust me. This also goes for those women (and teens) who think they need caffeine to get their day going. No one should "need" caffeine, ever. If you do, you'd better be asking why. Don't forget all the things caffeine does to your body and mind. Can you really tell me this is a healthy choice? (The 5 will definitely help control cravings for caffeine.)

I guess I should also be concerned about my kids drinking all those coffee drinks?

You should be very concerned. I'm astounded at how many teens, even young children, I see so often buying those highly caffeinated-chocolate-dripping-overflowing-whipped-cream drinks. *Are the parents not aware that caffeine is a drug?* The chocolate is another stimulant source. A double whammy. Add the milk with all that lactose, and the whipped cream. *Getting the picture?* Considering the latest craze is for high school, even middle school kids, to grab a flavored latte (averages 320 calories, 39g carbs/sugar) double espresso, or mocha mint frappuccino (390 calories, with a staggering 74g carbs/sugar) before and after school, the health issues with our youth will only get worse. I'm further dismayed that no one in the health industry is concerned by this fashionable trend. But now add the aforementioned concerns to the typical teenage diet of fast food and endless sodas, and well, it's no wonder our youth are so damn depressed, emotionally out of control, unable to concentrate, filled with rage, gaining fat at an alarming rate, anxious and—suicidal. Parents need to realize that caffeine, *no matter the source* (coffee, iced tea, chocolate, sodas, Red Bull-type energy drinks, etc.) deplete serotonin, causing cravings, eating disorders, weight gain, depression, agitation, anxiety, ADD/ADHD, and, yes, even suicidal thoughts.

Find the *underlying* cause of your illness.
Don't mask it with harmful drugs, as they will create new disease.

Oh, you're absolutely right. Is this why ADD/ADHD are so prevalent?
Yes, more often than not. Remember, when serotonin levels are depleted, among many things, our ability to concentrate is greatly affected. Rather than the medical industry wanting to find out the underlying cause of your in ability to focus, they'd much rather prescribe a drug. This is because the doctors don't make money by telling you to go home and reevaluate your eating habits and lifestyle. Yet this is where you will truly find quality of health. Instead, doctors eagerly prescribe a drug, which will, in turn, create new side effects, which will create yet another so-called illness, for which they will again eagerly prescribe yet another drug. It is a vicious and continuous cycle driven solely by greed.

What about the latest adult ADD?
Same thing. This is, pathetically, nothing more than the drug companies looking to expand their drug sales. After all, there are only so many children they can get on their drugs for ADD/ADHD. But by creating this new disease called "Adult ADD," they open the door to earn billions more. In reality, it is a *condition* that is due to low serotonin. And low serotonin is due to poor diet and lifestyle habits. Once again, it's important to realize that I have personally lived most of what I speak: mood swings, cravings, bloating, fat gain, etc. This is no different. Please allow me to share my personal experience with adult ADD: I've been taking the 5 for nearly six years. Except when I'm testing formulas, I'm never without it. Once years ago, while I was still writing my first book, did I actually experience the symptoms of what the medical industry has recently labeled, "Adult ADD."

I wrote most of that book in about 11 months. Because it's my passion, there was very little effort. It simply flowed. So much, in fact, that at times I would get up and review my work from the day before and not remember half the chapters that I had written. I'm not kidding. It was as if someone else had written them. Nevertheless, it was effortless. However, after I was off product for about a week, I was suddenly no longer able to concentrate. It was like a TV channel that kept switching. As hard as I tried, I couldn't stay focused. Thoughts were there one minute, gone the next. Hell, I couldn't even focus long enough to write one lousy sentence, let alone a chapter. I was stunned. Frustrated. I needed to finish my book, but it was hopeless, as I was unable to hold a thought long enough. I also found it all very telling.

Suddenly, I knew exactly what all those commercials about ADD, adult or otherwise, were talking about. But I also knew that by merely boosting and maintaining my serotonin, *minus any drugs*, my mind would once again be in total control, sharp, focused, and creative. And that is precisely what happened. Back on product and within only three doses, I wrote four new chapters in one afternoon. More importantly, it was, once again, effortless. My mind was sharp, focused, creatively driven, and long-lasting. What a huge difference.

That's amazing. Both my children and sister were diagnosed with ADD. Considering their horrendous diets, I'm quite sure this is the underlying cause. A healthier diet is a must. Now, as if I don't already know the answer, what are your thoughts on cigarettes? In addition to nicotine being a stimulant, it's a horrendously addictive and deadly product. Besides increasing your risks for heart disease, stroke, lung cancer, and sudden death, it will deplete serotonin, which will lead to numerous other health issues. Adults should not smoke, nor should our youth. Here's another flashback: Candy cigarettes. Ahhh, remember those? Back in the 1960s, they had names and packages that were nearly identical to the real thing. They were long, white candy sticks with tiny red tips. They were the ultimate in cool! Or so we thought. As a child, we used to love to pretend to be smoking. *How sick is that?* Only now, as I write this chapter, do I suddenly realize the dreadful marketing scheme that was behind these candy cigarettes. There's compelling evidence that the candy makers actually worked with the cigarette companies to attract young smokers. Little did we know, as children, what their motives were. Unfortunately, neither did most parents.

Isn't there a lot of peer pressure for kids?
Of course. Studies show that much younger kids are feeling the peer pressure to drink, smoke, take X (ecstasy), and have sex. Whether it's the "friends with benefits" type of sex or a serious relationship, it's way too much pressure and responsibility at that age. Sex and all the emotions, health risks, etc., are tough enough to deal with when you're an adult, let alone a teenager, and most certainly not at 10 and 12. And if you think for one second that I don't understand the insatiable desire to explore, be it sexually or with things that alter one's mind, well, I can assure you, you would be wrong. Very wrong.

In high school, I, along with my few close friends, drank alcohol, smoked dope, even occasionally snorted blow, ate shrooms, and dropped acid. As a rebel, and as a teenager struggling emotionally, I wanted to experiment. But I did these drugs *freely,* not because of peer pressure. To a greater extent, I was trying to escape the reality of my home life.

Furthermore, I was also, and still am, a very sexual being. Uninhibited. Eager to explore. More importantly, highly selective and protection was, and is, a must. But, up until about age 14, I was perfectly content with just racin' around on motorcycles, shootin' hoops, and playin' football with the boys. Shortly thereafter, however, things began to change. Boys, or should I say men no less than 5–10 years older, were suddenly my entire focus. So, you see, I, too, understand and appreciate the need, the *desire* to quench one's sexual thirst.

"Friends with Benefits"

The biggest difference between my generation and what's going on now is that whether or not we engaged in oral, vaginal, or anal sex, we didn't lie to ourselves; we knew it was S-E-X, and we didn't pretend to be virgins. Moreover, we became sexually active, because we thought we were "in love." Yet the young girls today freely admit they're using their bodies, *their sexual abilities*, to just be more popular with the boys. Not just with one or two guys, but many, from orgies, rainbow parties, to tossing salad, etc. Well, here's a rude awakening, girls: This is not the kind of popularity or reputation you want.

Furthermore, why would you ever let a boy use you like this? This is such a pathetic game, a game in which you're being made fools of. In case you're not aware, your value as a female is not measured by your body parts. You do not need to give a boy a handjob, blowjob, or any other sexual favor to be an appreciated, admired, and lovable human being. You are worth so much more than this. Take your power back. Rise above this selfish trend, and let the pretty boys do their own dirty work.

To those girls who will most certainly seek the sexual thrill, at least I hope that when you do explore, you'll engage in this emotionally, mentally, and physically risky behavior with your eyes wide open and making damn sure the boys are strapped up before they put it down. Getting pregnant will seem like nothing compared to being infected with HIV. Anal sex drastically increases this deadly risk. Don't forget, condoms fail far too often. (Equally, the boys, though few there may be, should not feel pressured into having sex.)

Most teens, including myself, also know the pain of losing a parent through divorce or another tragedy. This pain, this sense of loss, can be devastating. Now, combine that with the above, along with the normal hormonal changes that any teenager will experience, and, well, I hope you're starting to realize why they're so depressed, and why it's so critical for them to eat healthy and properly maintain their serotonin levels. Please help them eat a healthier diet before you put them on any pharmaceutical drugs.

What things should I cut out?
Cut out any and all sodas, fruit drinks, iced tea, and any other caffeinated beverages. This includes the many new, hip energy drinks that are loaded with sugar, caffeine, and

numerous other stimulants. Avoid alcohol, nicotine, chocolate, aspartame, high-fructose corn syrup, sugar, cereal, milk (especially fat free/skim milk), nachos, rice cakes, fast food, pasta, white bread, rice, potatoes, bagels, pizza, biscuits and gravy, fried food, etc. The list is endless. I think you have a good idea. Simply stated: You need to read the food labels. This alone will help you tremendously in selecting the right food for you and your family. Just remember, you need to eat real food, not processed or refined food. I know this will seem overwhelming at first, but your health and the health of your children depend on it. These are all healthy habits that you need to make part of your life starting now.

To reiterate, healthy levels of serotonin will help control the cravings for the carbs that spike insulin. And, because insulin is what causes the body to store fat, the less insulin spiking, the less fat stored. This same unhealthy food, however, also causes depression. Please understand that once you boost and maintain your serotonin, your mind will become quiet, the cravings will stop. You will no longer have the desire for those types of carbs/beverages. It will happen effortlessly. You will finally be free of those insatiable cravings and purported food addictions. Your mood will also become much more stable. You'll feel less anxious, less stressed, slower to anger. You'll be more focused and feel so much happier. You'll feel in control of your life once again.

I'm concerned about my son. What are the statistics on teens and depression?

I was stunned to discover that suicide is the third leading cause of death for teens. Each year, approximately 20% of all high school students think about committing suicide. 10% try. To reiterate, the antidepressants doctors are prescribing to these teens are actually causing *more* suicidal thoughts, even suicide itself. There is currently an investigation into these drugs. The drugs thought to be effective in treating children with major depression are themselves now being investigated as a possible cause of suicidal behavior. Numerous lawsuits have been filed against the makers of these drugs.

NEWS UPDATE: The medical industry came out in an attempt to defend their drugs and these latest charges. They're claiming that "because these kids are now able to 'talk about' their depression means that the drugs are, in fact, working. They see it as a positive sign that these kids are actually getting better." *Excuse me?* While I am not a medical doctor, I seriously doubt this rationalization. So should you. But hold on a second Let's be fair here. In the furthest stretch of one's imagination, let's say it's true. How, then, do they explain that during the clinical trials on these various antidepressant drugs, dozens of patients were not only experiencing suicidal thoughts, but many actually committed suicide? And under the FDA's very own analysis, there have been more than 20,000 Prozac-related suicides since 1987. Huh? *How do they rationalize that?* They can't. Chillingly, the FDA allows these DEADLY drugs to be marketed. *But why?* How can a drug be sold that causes the exact same deadly side effects that it's intended to be eliminating? *Where is the outrage by the parents and our government?* This all leaves me speechless.

NEWS UPDATE: As reported by CNN, the FDA has suddenly backed off its warning that antidepressants such as Zoloft, Paxil, and Prozac can cause suicidal actions among children and teens taking those drugs. Instead, the FDA, in a revised warning, changed the wording to state only that the drugs "increased the 'risk' of suicidal thinking and behavior in short-term studies of adolescents and children." Limiting their warning to a mere "risk," rather than admitting the drugs actually can *cause* suicidal behavior in younger patients, is a major and exceedingly disturbing retreat for the FDA. Do you want to know *why* the FDA backed down? Here's yet another contemptible example of the FDA being bought off by big pharma. The record is clear: They backed off after several months of lobbying by the pharmaceutical industry. *HELLO?!! Doesn't anyone find this alarming, let alone illegal?* I should hope so. They all need to be investigated before even more people die at their greedy, lying, manipulative hands.

I agree! Along with a healthier diet, aren't there safer ways to treat depression?

Yes, there are. Furthermore, I have <u>never</u> met anyone who was actually happy on an antidepressant. They were, though, numb, an emotionless zombie. Again, these drugs don't work. *Need more proof?* **MEDICAL UPDATE***:* "Two out of three people taking antidepressants still suffer with depression. Talk to your doctor today about adding Abilify." Big pharma's only solution is to take MORE DRUGS. Yet the following supplements have impressive studies supporting their ability to safely, and effectively, enhance serotonin.

5-HTP versus antidepressants:

Clinical studies indicate that 5-HTP is one of the safest, most effective methods of elevating serotonin, and, thus, treating depression. Unlike MAOIs (Monoamine Oxidase Inhibitors) such as Nardil, Parnate, etc., 5-HTP does not interfere with the activity of the enzyme that breaks down serotonin. Unlike SSRIs (Selective Serotonin Reuptake Inhibitors) such as Prozac, Zoloft, Paxil, etc., 5-HTP does not block reuptake of serotonin. 5-HTP is an amino acid. It does not interfere with the body's natural process of serotonin release, absorption, or elimination. It's safe, natural, affordable, non-habit-forming, exceptionally effective, works much faster than drugs, and no prescription is required. (5-HTP is my number one choice for elevating, and maintaining, serotonin.)

WARNING: Taking the 5, or any supp that enhances serotonin, in conjunction with antidepressants, is not recommended. The risk is called "serotonin syndrome." There's a very precise protocol. Before attempting to wean yourself off the drugs, learn how to eat healthy, stop consuming all the things that deplete serotonin. Next, tell your doctor your desires. (NOTE: I've weaned countless clients off these drugs—and alleviated their depression. I offer private consults/programs, with 100% success rate.)

NEWS UPDATE: Actor Jim Carrey spoke openly about his bouts with depression, issues with Prozac, and how he's come to learn how our diet plays a critical role in our mental health. He also talked about the "antidepressant supplements" he takes. You guessed it; 5-HTP. Like me, Jim now realizes there's a *cure* for depression. Bottom line, you have to be willing to live a healthy lifestyle. Then, watch how great you will feel!

A personal reflection . . .

With all this talk of depression, I feel the need to share my own personal story, as it may help you, or your teen. I feel it's paramount that you know that I speak not just as a researcher, but also as someone who has experienced what I write about. Obviously, by now, you know that I'm not pretending to be some sort of angel or puritan. Nor did I ever do anything based on peer pressure. That being said, throughout my late teens and into my early thirties, I loved going out, most often alone, and the edgier the place, the better. For me, that included going to clubs, dancing, drinking alcohol, and a few other party favors. But I still did my best to eat healthy and exercise regularly. I was fortunate to maintain my physique, while enjoying a few less than desirable habits. For me, it was all about balance and moderation, with an occasional escape from reality. Nevertheless, as time went on, alcohol no longer gave me the same pleasure it once did. I wasn't going out nearly as often as years prior, but when I did, I drank more than I should, I started to have blackouts, hangovers were pure hell, and even after the hangovers finally subsided, my mood would be altered for days. Hence, I cut back even more. But, still I found myself feeling emotionally weak, not my usual strong, carefree self. My tears fell quicker and more frequently. I also craved carbs, anything from subs, cereal, pretzels and pasta, carbs that I would normally never care for, were suddenly my only desire. (Considering I was years away from discovering serotonin, my only concern at that time was finding out why I felt so sad after a few lousy cocktails.)

I wrote my mood swings off to simply being hormonal, financial stress, boyfriend issues, all those things people at my age worried about. Although I'm blessed with the most won-derful friends, I've always been content in my time alone. It was at those sad times that I would find solace in working out and writing poetry. Not rhyming type of poetry, rather free-flowing-let-your-mind-run-wild kind of poetry. I had to write; it was my only way of releasing all that I felt. I never felt suicidal, but I definitely felt lost. Hopeless. Desperately alone in the world. And that is a terrible place to be. (On a very personal note, I also feared that I had possibly followed in my mother's footsteps. She had, sadly, been diagnosed with so-called "mental illness" many years prior.)

Ever since I was 15, writing had been my chosen therapy. Bob (aka Coach) Grimes, my high school creative writing teacher, was truly an amazing man, a man who inspired me in many ways, but he also insisted I keep a journal, a journal that was a safe haven for me to pour forth all that I was feeling. Right or wrong, I would never be judged. It was through this writing process (along with his genuine compassion) that I was able to mentally and emotionally survive those tormented teenage years. Ironically, years later, I discovered that my writing was, once again, the venue I chose to express my grief, my darkest fears, my overwhelming sense of foreboding that would unexpectedly envelope me. Writing allowed me to do this privately, without shame or judgment. Then, come the next morning, I felt fine. Life went on. Happily. Until I drank again. I still have those writings. It's rather sad to see just how dark my mood was.

As for my high school journals, my stepmother found them and was horrified by what she read. I can't recall exactly what I wrote, but whatever pain she felt when reading them, couldn't possibly compare to the pain I felt when writing them. To my grave disappointment, she threw them away. With regard to my drinking, I continued on this unhealthy path for years to come. To be honest, I assumed it was just who I was. Too emotional. Too sensitive. The fact of the matter was, my mental state of mind had nothing to do with my mother's illness or with me being too emotional. These mood swings were, without a doubt, directly linked to the alcohol.

Why didn't you stop?

Why? Good question. I suppose I didn't really want to stop. I loved going out. As a single woman with a very adventurous spirit, I enjoyed meeting new people, and going to nightclubs and intimate wine bars was the way I preferred to socialize. However, and more importantly, it was actually that quiet, but oh, so powerful little voice within, that voice we now know as a craving, that kept me coming back for more. No matter how bad I felt, it all seemed worth it. Little did I know it was just another craving. After all, alcohol is primarily sugar, and it's recognized by the body as sugar. This craving is no different from the cravings you get for bread, candy, chips, or soda. FACT: Alcohol is made from either grain or fruit, both of which are carbohydrates. Alcohol is a combination of alcohol and sugar. Alcohol will, hence, have the same effect on brain chemistry as the high GI carbs we've discussed. You drink it. Insulin is spiked. Insulin leads to serotonin elevation. Between the alcohol and the shift in brain chemistry, you start to feel good. Really good. And whoever stops at one drink? Regardless, the next day, you're undeniably serotonin deficient. Your brain then shifts to another type of carb that will once again trigger the release of this blissful, mood-altering brain chemical. This is exactly why after a night of partying you'll find yourself craving things like bagels, fries, pizza, chips, sodas, tacos, caffeine, or maybe even another cocktail. It is your brain merely trying once again to stimulate the production of serotonin. It is a cycle. Once you're aware of this cycle, this pattern of cravings, whether it's for alcohol or junk food, you'll hopefully be able to take control of these bad habits.

And your depressive moods?

Although alcohol first triggers the production of serotonin, it also depletes it. After a night of partying, my serotonin would plummet. This caused not only food cravings, but also mood swings. Some days, these mood swings plummeted to depression. *"Depression?"* What the hell did I know about depression? I just felt blue. Or so I believed. It is only now, after I've spent numerous years researching serotonin and its essential role in our physical, mental, and emotional health, that I can reflect and honestly understand what was happening to me. By sharing this story, *the direct relation to alcohol and depression,* I sincerely hope it helps save you, and others, from this senseless, self-inflicted emotional trauma.

How did you eventually stop?

I had no choice but to start listening to my body, as it was certainly letting me know that alcohol was not good for me, in many ways. Over the years, I had drastically cut back.

Since I began this journey, even one drink a month became too much for me. After about seven months of being on the 5, it amazingly squelched all desire for alcohol. Where I used to have my Thursday night urge to go out, craving a dirty martini in some soulful Ebony underground club, I now have no desire to drink. Best of all, I don't miss it. I feel wonderful without it. My moods are much more stable. I no longer suffer from those dark days. I haven't felt the need to write poetry in over 30 years. And I've stopped wasting time nursing hangovers. Maintaining my serotonin has given me far more than a leaner, healthier body. It has literally saved my life by keeping me from abusing my body and mind any further with this intoxicating, yet potentially dangerous toxin.

How does this happen?
Serotonin helps control carb/sugar cravings. Alcohol is made from either grain or fruit, both carbs. Don't forget that most people like to mix their preferred alcohol with some sort of soda, fruit juice, etc., which adds even more sugar, plus caffeine. All of these will further deplete serotonin. So you see, my desire for alcohol was the same as someone craving a chocolate bar or a bowl of cereal. The brain exhibits low serotonin in many different ways, and it will continually make you want the things it knows will elevate this brain chemical. Without a doubt, my brain knew that alcohol would elevate my serotonin.

It's not like I drink that much. Are you saying I should quit altogether?
Yes, I am. Look at all the side effects alcohol has on your health, on your life. However, it's up to you on how you choose to use the information. Over the years of training clients, I've had many who expect me to give them a perfect body, while they ignore all the things I teach them regarding diet, alcohol, caffeine, and many other health concerns. While I'm more than confident in my abilities, I'm not a magician. I need their help once they leave the studio. You need to realize that if you're truly serious about losing excess body fat, lowering blood pressure, alleviating depression, etc., alcohol is something you need to avoid. Alcohol is a leading contributor to hypertension and depression. Alcohol triggers insulin, thereby, causing the production of harmful cholesterol. High levels of insulin also fuel cancer cells.

MEDICAL UPDATE: Research now shows that drinking just 1 to 2 drinks a day increases a woman's risk of breast cancer by 10%) Alcohol depletes serotonin, which leads to numerous health issues including PMS, ADD, rage, insomnia, low sex drive, body pain, carb/sugar cravings, weight gain, depression, and anxiety. Many of those who drink, also don't realize that their body has to first burn off the alcohol before it will start to burn their stored fat. Alcohol is nothing more than useless calories and a momentary break from reality. I admit we all certainly need a break from reality now and then, however, you need to look at the bigger picture and see the effects alcohol has on your life. I've personally seen a huge change in my body (and emotions) since I stopped drinking. (The 5 will help control these cravings, but if someone doesn't make the effort, no amount of working out or product will help them. You have to be willing. You have to make the effort.)

What do you suggest?

Start by getting on a quality 5-HTP. I also respectfully insist that, for the first 90 days of this new healthy lifestyle, you avoid all alcohol for the reasons just mentioned. Allow yourself to really get into a healthy workout routine and eating program. Give yourself three months of feeling what it's like to just focus on being healthy. Your body composition will start to change. Toxins will flush out of your system. Your mind will become clearer, more focused. Your emotions will be far more stable. You'll start to feel a difference in all aspects of your life. You'll be astonished at just how good you can really feel without all the poisons that come from alcohol, processed food, etc. My personal guarantee: If you devote three unadulterated months to this healthy lifestyle, I guarantee you will not want to go back to your old habits. You will feel so much happier, healthier, stronger and more self-confident, and all of this combined, will motivate you to continue on this path. The sense of pride you will feel for having accomplished this lifelong goal is enough to inspire you to take it even further. You will be amazed at what you can create with your body. But know this, your goal is simple: Do not let yourself get overwhelmed by looking too far down the proverbial road. Simply focus on one week at a time. Each passing week will bring even more exciting changes in both your body and mind. Once again motivating you to take it further. Your success will equally inspire others around you.

But isn't there pressure to drink when you go out on a date or with friends?

First of all, I rarely dated. When I did, the man respected my decision, especially after I told him why I no longer drank. As for my friends, likewise. Please understand that I'm fine with those who drink. We make our own choices. It's simply my choice now not to. The reward: I'm a sober, safe driver, no risk of DUIs or harming another. (I'm also much better prepared to drive defensively.) Come the next day, I wake up bright and early with no headache, no hangover, no regrets, sexual or otherwise. I'm ready to work out, run my dogs, go to the beach, anything to enjoy the day. I must be honest, sex has never been better since I quit drinking. I think many of us are used to being intimate with the help of some sort of mind-altering substance, alcohol being the most common, that we forget where such intense passion can truly take our body and mind. (With the right lover, of course.) Furthermore, avoiding alcohol makes it a lot easier to maintain a lean, healthy body since I don't trigger cravings. My moods are also much more stable. I'm less emotional, less stressed, and less anxious.

I'm ready to quit drinking after that! What about the elderly and drinking?

This is a serious issue. Researchers are now calling this phenomenon "Late-Onset Alcoholism." In one clinical study, 41% of the people age 65 and over who were enrolled in an alcohol treatment program, reported that their alcohol problems began after age 60. Most seniors who do have an alcohol problem are unable or unwilling to recognize it. Others simply can't recognize it because of cognitive impairment caused by the alcohol.

I worry that my mother drinks too much. But what can I do?

I know this is a very sensitive and personal matter. Nonetheless, my suggestion is to first talk to her, compassionately. Tell her your concerns. If she is open, then start with her diet. Use the information you've learned here and put it to work. Next, get her on the 5. This will help her control the alcohol cravings. You must understand that both changing her diet and using any such product will require time, effort, and tremendous patience before you start to see a shift in her behavior. (Caffeine is also a concern, as it's depleting her serotonin, thereby, perpetuating her cravings for sugar, i.e., alcohol.) If your mother chooses to ignore you, you'll at least know that you made an honest and loving attempt to help her. And, while you may have nothing but good intentions, we each have to live our own life. Your mother has the right to do with her life as she wishes, just as you do with yours. If she chooses to drink, in excess or otherwise, it's her choice. It won't be easy to watch, but it's not your life. Be there for her, but without contributing to her drinking lifestyle. Your teenage son, however, is a different story. He is your son and living under your care. You need to do whatever it takes to help him.

Amazing! I certainly relate to the senseless hangovers, depression and anxiety. My son is often depressed after a night out with his friends. I'll do everything I can to help him improve his health through a healthy diet <u>before</u> I put him on any drugs.
I'm sure you can understand my extreme frustration when I see the endless drug commercials marketing their antidepressants. With regard to teens, considering their horrendous high-sugar diets, along with drinking, smoking, takin' X, hormone shifts, and the stress of just being that age, it's no wonder they're depressed, even suicidal. Their serotonin is frighteningly depleted. But you have choices. Please keep those many choices in mind before you put your family or yourself on any pharmaceutical drugs.

BTW: For those parents who aren't aware, ecstasy (X) and/or Molly works primarily by flooding the body with serotonin. Some teens are hip enough, though, to take the 5 to help avoid the depression that most often follows after partying. Now, if you could only get them to take the 5, <u>minus</u> the X, you'd see so many wonderful changes in them.

ECSTASY: Personally, I question the many professed risks of taking X, as I think the real danger comes from the hazardous drugs and chemical compounds that X is often cut with. Nonetheless, even if the risks are real, why then, are alcohol and cigarettes—two products that have long been proven to be addictive and deadly—legal and so heavily promoted? Easy answer: Big business. Bigger profits.

To be perfectly honest, of all the drugs I've tried, X was the most amazing high. It's a drug that makes you see only good in others and opens you up to such deep and honest emotions. It's a drug that is simply about love. No anger. No animosity. Just love. It is a drug, that if produced safely, has the potential to literally end racism and religious wars worldwide, and, put every struggling marriage/relationship back together.

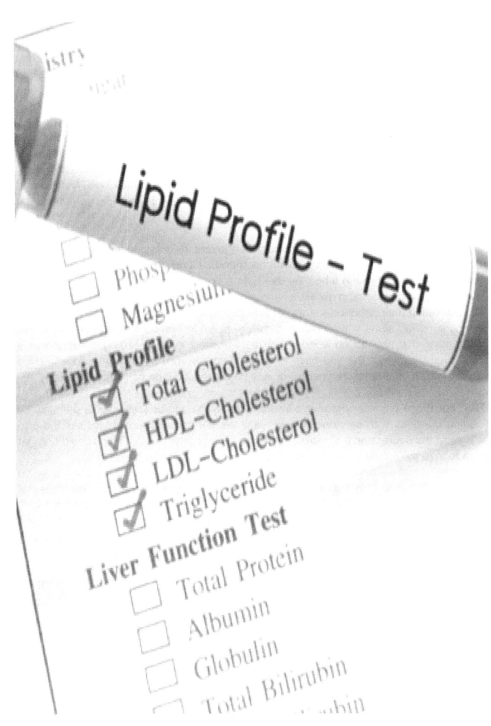

19

INSULIN & HOW IT AFFECTS CHOLESTEROL
Avoid junk carbs, instead, eat healthy fat and cholesterol

ATTENTION READER: Please take this chapter very seriously. Stop risking your life with statins. This is the #1 concern for people over 40. But you have to know "what to eat," so you can alleviate your cholesterol concerns—and live a much longer, healthier life. I deal with this issue with most of my clients. Yet with every client, as I bring their body fat down with proper nutrition, I equally redirect their lipids in exactly the direction that will help reduce their risks for heart disease, heart attack, stroke, dementia, and more.

Dementia?
Yes, dementia. The brain is approximately 60-70% fat and 25% cholesterol. It is the most cholesterol-rich organ in the body. Our brain *thrives* on fat and cholesterol. I warn my clients about this all the time. Johns Hopkins researchers now believe Alzheimer's is due the increase of statins—and to low serotonin. I agree, because serotonin is the master communicator among all brain chemicals—and because low serotonin pushes us toward unhealthy lifestyle habits. If we can destroy our heart, kidneys, liver, bones, etc., with unhealthy food/drink, why would our brain be any different? Trust me, it's not.

I'm impressed! I hear all the warnings about cholesterol, but I'm not sure what it is.
Most do not. Many also fear it, when they should not. Cholesterol is a soft, waxy, fat-like substance found in the bloodstream and in all of our cells. We need cholesterol. It's a vital part of being healthy. Cholesterol helps produce cell membranes, provides structure within cell membranes and keeps those cells permeable. Several of our major hormones (DHEA, cortisol, testosterone, estradiol, progesterone and vitamin D), are all made from cholesterol. Cholesterol provides a type of insulation around nerves, allowing electrical impulses to move freely. Neurotransmitters are dependent on cholesterol, therefore, necessary for proper brain function. Cholesterol and other fats are water insoluble, i.e., they cannot dissolve in the bloodstream. They have to be transported to/from the cells by special carriers known as lipoproteins. Please read the following with great care. Learn how to interpret your lipid profile. It could literally save your life.

TOTAL CHOLESTEROL: (TC) is NOT an accurate way to asses one's risks for heart disease. It's a useless number, but one that most doctors, unfortunately, focus on so as to sell you a deadly statin. My TC and your TC could be the same, but the numbers used to add up and provide the TC, would be entirely different.

HDL: High-density lipoprotein, the so-called good cholesterol. Most HDL is made by the liver. HDL carries cholesterol away from the parts of the body that no longer need it and sends it back to the liver for storage. High blood levels of HDL can reduce risk of heart disease. The higher the number, the better. FACT: The leaner your stomach, the lower your body fat = higher HDL, lower VLDL, LDL, and trigs, the lower your health risks. Your goal? 70>.

LDL: Low-density lipoprotein, the so-called bad cholesterol. This is what the AMA/FDA claims causes heart disease. However, the science behind that claim is non-existent. LDL repairs and rebuilds. It also delivers cholesterol to the brain. The brain thrives on cholesterol! FACT: The bigger your stomach, the higher your body fat = higher LDL, VLDL, and trigs, with lower HDL, the greater your health risks.

WARNING: When you get your cholesterol checked, look for "calc" after your LDL score. That calc stands for "calculated." It's a cheaper method in which to calculate your LDL. But guess what? That LDL number will always be *higher*. How convenient. Just another way to scare you into taking a deadly statin. I don't give a damn about my LDL. I focus on keeping my trigs low and HDL high. They're the most important. Again, the less insulin you trigger, the lower your body fat, the healthier your lipids will be.

VLDL: Very low-density lipoprotein. VLDL contain high amounts of triglycerides, with very little protein. VLDL are your trigs divided by 5. The lower, the better. FACT: The bigger your stomach, the higher your body fat = higher VLDL, LDL, and trigs, with lower HDL, the greater your health risks.

TRIGLYCERIDES: This, is what I care about most. Triglycerides are a type of fat found in the blood. When you eat too many and/or unhealthy carbs/sugar, your body will convert them into triglycerides, i.e., body fat. FACT: The bigger your stomach, the higher your body fat = higher trigs, LDL and VLDL, with lower HDL, the higher your health risks. Your goal? Aim for 40-60, nowhere near "up to 149" that the AMA considers healthy.

The best way to achieve healthy levels of these lipids, thereby, reducing your health risks, is by living a healthy lifestyle. This healthy lifestyle will help you decrease trigs, LDL and VLDL, while raising your HDL. Furthermore, being healthy and/or having risk factors, goes well beyond a lipid profile.

Once again, please focus on trigs and HDL; getting trigs 40-60, with HDL 70+, while, reducing your insulin gauge (widest girth of stomach). When I reduce a client's stomach, trigs drop and HDL rises. Science. Get your stomach down by eating, as I suggest, use the 5 to maintain your serotonin and insulin levels, and your lipids will go in the right direction.

Okay great! How does one get cholesterol?
Our liver makes it. We also get it from the food we eat, which I highly recommend. Contrary to what most experts will tell you, *you need to eat healthy food rich in cholesterol to shut*

down your body's internal clock and keep it from producing its own. If you deprive your body of this vital nutrient, your body will be forced to produce its own. To avoid this health risk, you need to eat food (at every meal) that contains cholesterol. If you don't, your body will make cholesterol from carbs; through the insulin spiking process. This will elevate your LDL, and lower your HDL. Excellent sources of cholesterol-laden food: Red meat, shellfish, butter, poultry, fish, cream, ghee, cheese and eggs.

Eggs? I thought eggs were bad for us?
This scare tactic was perpetuated over 50 years ago by the cereal industry and now by big pharma. (And, no, eating Cherrios will <u>not</u> lower your cholesterol.) Eggs are a perfect pro-tein, a healthy source of cholesterol—and THE MOST perfect food. They're low in calories and sodium, just .6g carbs per egg, an excellent source of complete protein, exceptional fat and cholesterol. In addition, eggs contain a wonderful abundance of vitamins and min-erals. With all these many benefits, how can eggs possibly be bad for us?

What is the connection between insulin and cholesterol?
Anything that triggers insulin <u>increases</u> the overproduction of cholesterol. This list includes sugar, stress, alcohol, prescription and nonprescription drugs, OTC meds, poor diet, low fat/low calorie diets, cigarettes, lack of healthy fats and proteins, caffeine, ma huang, all stimulants, processed and refined food, a sedentary lifestyle, excessive, and high GI carb intake equals high insulin levels, which creates the most harmful form of cholesterol. This is what increases your risks for heart disease, heart attack, stroke, dementia, etc.

Will the 5 also help control insulin levels?
Correct. Because the 5 will help you greatly reduce your intake of the type of carbs that trigger insulin. But the key to a healthy cholesterol panel is to live a healthy *lifestyle*. It is <u>not</u> just about a number. You need to do what it takes to stabilize your insulin.

<u>FACT</u>: A majority of people with alleged high cholesterol *never* suffer heart attacks.
<u>FACT</u>: More than 60% of all heart attacks and strokes occur in people with so-called *nor-mal* cholesterol panels.

How do you feel about the latest change in guidelines for "total" cholesterol?
When the medical industry, i.e., the drug companies, changed the cholesterol guidelines from 220 to 200mg/dL (recently even as low as 180), the number of people who were suddenly "sick or at risk" tripled. Literally overnight, 104 million Americans were scared into believing they had to be on these drugs! This alone increased cholesterol drug sales by over an astounding 32%, earning the drug companies over $12.5 billion. If that wasn't enough, the NCEP (National Cholesterol Education Program) suggested that the new guidelines for LDL be lowered from 130 to 100mg/dL or less. Those considered high risk should aim for <70. This suggestion was based on clinical studies performed by who else, *the drug companies.* Not to mention, the NCEP works hand in hand with the FDA.

My first reaction to this latest change was, "When will it ever end? This means the drug companies basically want every single adult on their lifelong, cholesterol-lowering drugs." This will create billions in new revenue for the pharmaceutical companies. Lowering their guidelines will have an astronomical effect on millions of people who will be scared into believing they must be on these drugs. There are over 60 million people on some sort of statin. This new guideline will push the number to over 100 million! I guarantee you that most people will, unfortunately, never even question this. This tactic is outrageous and again based on the greed of big pharma.

What are these drugs designed to do?
These drugs, called statins, are HMG-CoA reductase inhibitors. They were designed to inhibit the production of cholesterol, primarily to help lower TC (Total Cholesterol) and LDL levels. Yet they do nothing to help raise the protective HDL levels or lower harmful trigs, which are my primary focus. The proposed goal of these statin drugs: To help prevent coronary heart disease. However, this is absolute BS. These statin drugs, like most other pharma drugs, are not what the medical industry claims. Furthermore, serious consideration should be given to this recent report: "Nine statins, commonly used at a dose to lower TC to <160mg/dL, are associated with higher cancer rates."

Cancer? I'm afraid to ask, but are there any other side effects?
Yes, there are literally dozens of other serious health risks to consider. Researchers from the U.S. National Institutes of Health found that the use of cholesterol-lowering drugs during the first trimester of pregnancy is associated with limb deformities and severe central nervous system defects. These medical findings were published in a research letter in the *New England Journal of Medicine*. It disclosed that 20 of 52 babies exposed to these drugs in the womb were born with malformations. And 1 to 3% of the prescriptions for these medications are for women in their childbearing years. Lipitor, Zocor, Pravachol, Crestor, Lescol, Mevacor, and Baycol were all linked to these studies.

Anything else to watch for?
Plenty. Other side effects reported range from constipation, myopathy, polyneuropathy, myalgia, liver and kidney damage, amnesia, and congestive heart failure. *All of this for drugs that do NOT work.* CNN reported that statin drugs were known to cause nerve damage in one in every 2,200 patients. For those over 50 and on the drugs for over two years, the chances of nerve damage were 26 times higher than for the normal population. That puts over 6,000 people at risk for nerve damage each year. (Sadly, my own father refused to put his statin down. He died due to kidney failure.) With regard to the brain and central nervous system side effects, a separate study showed that 100% of the participants, after only six months on the statin drugs, suffered measurable declines in cognition. To avoid these deadly drugs, you need to take a much closer look at your diet and lifestyle, then make the necessary changes starting today.

Furthermore, if statins really are the "miracle drugs" that the drug industry would like us to believe they are, *why* then are more people than ever before dying of heart failure? *Why?* Because these statin drugs are doing nothing to help prevent heart attacks, they are instead, at the very least, dangerously affecting your liver's ability to make CoQ10 (coenzyme Q10), a substance found in most tissues in the body and in some food. It's an antioxidant and used by the body to produce energy for cells. Without CoQ10, the cells in your muscles can't produce enough energy. Subsequently, these muscles weaken dramatically. The heart just happens to be one of these muscles. See my concern?

To reiterate, make the much-needed changes in your diet and overall lifestyle. Research. Educate yourself about your options. Avoid anything that triggers insulin. This includes, but is not limited to, alcohol, caffeine, nicotine, sugar, high GI carbs, excess of carbs, processed/refined food, etc. Eat a diet rich in healthy fats and cholesterol. It may not be easy in the beginning, but maintaining healthy serotonin levels will control your cravings. Controlling your cravings will help stabilize your insulin. Start some sort of exercise program. You need to be devoted to this if you really want to make changes. It's possible to turn your health around by making better, healthier choices. Don't cheat yourself or your loved ones. After six months, go back to your doctor and ask her (or him) to run the *appropriate* test, the test that will determine whether or not your arteries are clogged. After all, this is what causes heart disease. Please understand that you can reverse many of these health problems without having to risk your life by using drugs. Not only do these drugs merely mask symptoms, they inevitably come with serious, if not, life-threatening side effects. These drugs, will, undoubtedly cause new diseases/illnesses. Is it worth it?

FACT: Cholesterol does NOT cause heart disease. Heart disease, heart attack, and stroke are caused by plaquing of the arteries, which is caused by high insulin levels. Avoid anything that causes insulin levels to spike, especially long-term.

<u>MEDICAL NEWS</u>: From the American Academy of Pediatrics, "Doctors should measure cholesterol concentrations in children aged two years and over and should treat them with high concentrations of statins, probably for life." Equally disturbing, this report echoed last year's report by the AMA.

<u>PERSONAL UPDATE</u>: I've touted the health benefits of eating healthy fat and cholesterol, be it eggs, butter, shellfish, poultry, organ meats, fish, heavy cream, cheese, and sardines for years. At 62 years of age, here are my numbers: HDL 77, range 45+ / Trigs 40, range 0-149 / VLDL 8, range 5-40 / LDL 130, range 0-99. Waist 26" / Body fat 13% / Weight 130 lbs. Because my HDL, VLDL, trigs, body fat and waist circumference are all excellent, and because we are far more than just these numbers, I'm not worried about my so-called high LDL. That's not my concern. Not at all. Rather, it's about a healthy lifestyle, keeping my trigs and body fat low, with high HDL.

Need further inspiration? I recently had, not one, but three separate medical doctors say to me, "I wish my lipids were as good as yours!" I modestly handed them my business card.

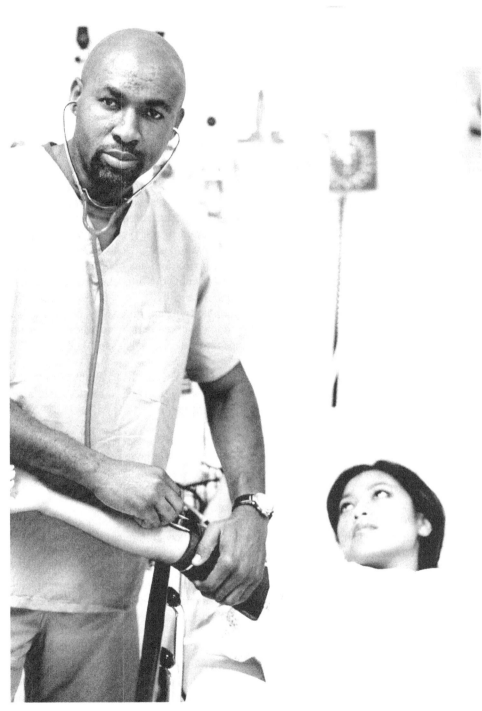

20

INSULIN & HOW IT AFFECTS
BLOOD PRESSURE

How do high insulin levels affect blood pressure?
First, allow me to say that those with high blood pressure have a much higher risk of getting heart disease. High blood pressure can be caused by several factors, but my focus is on those related to "high insulin" levels. High insulin levels can affect blood pressure in two ways:

1) Insulin promotes an abnormal increase of salt retention. The kidneys are responsible for regulating sodium levels in the blood, but this salt increase leads to water retention. This higher fluid levels may cause high blood pressure.

2) Insulin excites the nervous system. This increases the amount of blood being pumped out with every contraction of the heart. Not only will this cause high blood pressure, but it will also lead to stiffer, less pliable artery walls. This can lead to heart damage, a heart attack, even sudden death.

What exactly is sodium?
Sodium is a mineral that the body requires, but in small amounts. We don't want just sodium. We also need the 60+ other trace minterals. Read your food/drink labels and watch for the name "sodium chloride." (Sodium chloride is another name for table salt.)

Does table salt contribute to high blood pressure?
Yes, because it's highly processed and stripped of other vital minerals. Please avoid. * (See below.) Understand, though, you do not have to actually add salt to your food to be eating too much salt. Once again, read the nutrition facts label to see how much sodium is in the food you eat. Food to watch out for are all processed food, soups (canned and freshly made), snack food, crackers, condiments (mustard, ketchup, dressings, relish, soy sauce, etc.) smoked, salted, pickled, canned fish, meats and vegetables, processed cheese, etc.

How much sodium do I need each day?
The body needs, at minimum, 500 milligrams of sodium daily. However, most experts agree that sodium intake should be around 2,300mg per day for healthy adults. * **NOTE:** When eating based on this far healthier lifestyle, you'll need 2,000 to 4,000mg.

How will the 5 help control insulin levels?
The 5 will help control the cravings for the countless high GI carbs/beverages that spike

In addition to high blood pressure, a build-up of sodium in the body can cause thirst, water retention, and shortness of breath. This can greatly increase your risk of a stroke or heart attack. (One teaspoon of salt = 2,000mg of sodium. Use Redmond Real Sea Salt instead, because, once again, our body needs the 60+ other trace minerals, too.

What is considered to be a normal, healthy blood pressure?

Excellent question, considering that after the drug companies saw such a profitable response when they lowered cholesterol guidelines, they wasted no time in doing the same thing with blood pressure guidelines. Not so long ago, normal BP was 140/90. Suddenly 115/70 is considered a risk for stroke or heart attack. Doesn't anyone question their motives here? Why doesn't anyone demand explanations for this drastic and terribly convenient change?

To truly determine your blood pressure, it should be taken on at least three separate occasions. Take it when you're rested and calm—not in the busy, stressful part of your day. Blood pressure can also vary 5 to 30 points within seconds. The top number can be anywhere from 90–240, and the bottom number can be anywhere from 60–140. Blood pressure is measured in millimeters of mercury, which is written down as: mmHg. The following is a range from optimal to high. My BP runs 100/60, HR 40-45.

Optimal BP: Less than 120/over less than 80
Pre-hypertension: 120–130/over 80–89
High–normal BP: 130–139/over 89
High BP: 140+/over 90+
Optimal Heart Rate (18 and older): 60–100 beats per minute

What do the numbers actually represent?

There are two components of a blood pressure reading. Example: 115/65. The top number, 115, is the systolic pressure. This is the blood pressure in the arteries when the heart is pumping blood. The bottom number, 65, is the diastolic pressure. It represents the pressure in the arteries when the heart is resting and filling with blood. As this can be rather confusing, one more time: The systolic pressure shows the pressure in your arteries when your heart is forcing blood through them. The diastolic pressure shows the pressure in your arteries when your heart relaxes.

FOR AN ACCURATE BLOOD PRESSURE READING:

When you see your doctor, don't let them take your BP the minute you get into the room, because your BP will vary 5 to 30+ points within seconds. Plus, some people have "white coat" syndrome, which will drive it up, as well. So, relax. Breathe deep. Politely insist that they take it correctly. Unfortunately, very few do. One nurse wanted to take my BP over my wool jacket and with my arm hanging straight down. I insisted she do it right. She got angry. Too bad. CORRECT WAY: Your arm needs to be held up at heart level, fully extended, no bend, and resting on something, with your feet on the ground, and with an empty insulin levels. However, high GI carbs are found in most processed/snack food, i.e., pretzels, chips, crackers, etc. This same food is often excessively high in sodium. A double whammy, as high sodium also leads to high insulin levels. The 5 will, though, by controlling your cravings for junk food, inadvertently control your intake of this high sodium food.

The 5 will also help you avoid alcohol, caffeine and nicotine. Each of these lead to high insulin levels. The 5 will help reduce stress and anxiety. Both equally lead to high insulin levels. The 5 will help you live a far healthier lifestyle, which includes regular exercise. Insulin levels will, subsequently, become much more stable. Again, do whatever it takes to avoid spiking your insulin, especially over an extended period of time.

MAGNESIUM, THE MIRACLE MINERAL:

Magnesium is one of the most important minerals you're most certainly not getting enough of in your diet. Besides being a major contributor in over 325 enzyme systems throughout the body, magnesium is also essential for achieving and maintaining strong bones, restful sleep, regular bowels, healthy heart and blood pressure, and optimal brain function. Helps alleviate anxiety, too. These are just a few of the many reasons why so many health experts now refer to it as the "miracle" mineral.

There are numerous health conditions that can arise from magnesium deficiency, from migraines, hypertension, muscle cramps, to agitation, depression, anxiety, insomnia, diabetes, respiratory illnesses, and brain disorders. Vital organs, like the kidneys and gallbladder, rely on magnesium for proper function. Not a single system in the body is capable of working, as it should, without magnesium. It's critical to get enough of magnesium in your diet to avoid developing various diseases, as you age.

NOTE: All forms of magnesium are not created equal. Each form serves a different purpose. Research. Find which one you need. I use "NOW," a blend of malate, glycinate and citrate. Avoid oxide, as it's useless. If you're on a BP drug, monitor your BP closely, as the magnesium may bring it down quite fast. Next, be sure to eat a diet rich in potassium. Certain leafy greens, veggies, dairy, poultry, and fish can be rich in potassium. 1 cup cooked spinach = 840mg. Brussel sprouts = 504mg. Salmon = 719mg.

Typical range for magnesium is 100mg - 400mg. Start with 100mg. This is a beginner dose. With the brand I use above, I take 1 capsule in AM/1 capsule at PM. Most effective on an empty stomach. Increase slowly. If you get loose bowels, you're at your limit. Pull back slightly.

Finally, be sure to drink enough water. No one does. I've helped many clients get off hypertension meds (and alleviate their anxiety, myself included), with just the right dose and form of magnesium, plenty of water, and eating healthy with the help of the 5.

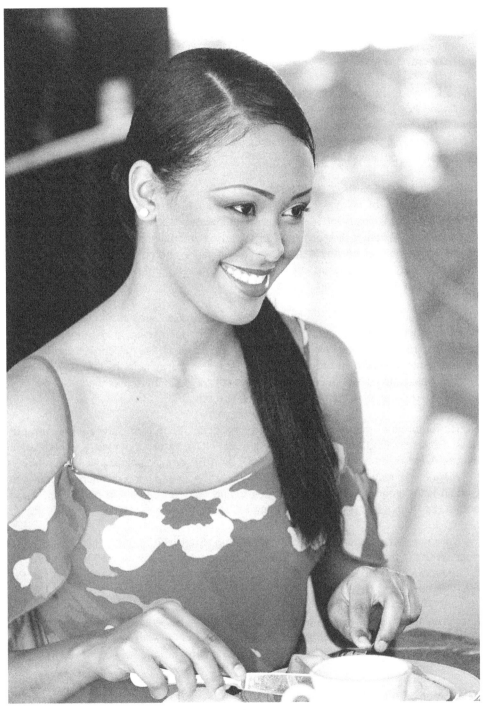

21

EATING HEALTHY
WITHOUT EVER FEELING DEPRIVED

Are you saying you never feel deprived?
That's exactly what I'm saying. To reiterate, life is <u>not</u> about living like a monk. Life is to be enjoyed in many delightful ways. Food just happens to be a small part of that. Although food can be absolutely divine, especially during the holidays, with family, sharing an intimate evening with someone special, or just a quiet meal alone, food stimulates a lot more than just our appetite. It also creates wonderful memories. Above all, food is fuel for our body. It is necessary for survival. Just please don't obsess about it.

So, do I eat healthy all the time? 99% of the time, I eat remarkably healthy, and what's more amazing, considering how stressed my life is, I can do so without any effort. I may occasionally want something I wouldn't necessarily recommend to my clients, but there isn't any effort to eating healthy, and I never have any sense of feeling hungry or deprived <u>if</u> I maintain my serotonin. Again, S-E-R-O-T-O-N-I-N is the key. I'm able to eat plenty of delicious food, combining healthy fats and proteins, with low GI, non-starchy carbs, while maintaining a lean, strong, and healthy physique.

The fact of the matter is, we are all creatures of habit. To achieve optimum health, we must learn (and be willing) to exchange the bad habits for healthier ones; that includes not skipping meals. I realize that, after nearly 50 years of being told "not to eat fat," there will be an adjustment. But, believe me, eating healthy fat does NOT make you fat. It is eating the *wrong* type of carbs (along with eating damaged fats that are found in junk/processed/fast food) that has caused the alarming rate of obesity in this country.

Okay, so what should I eat?
Eat balanced, nutritious meals. Combine food groups, eating quality protein, healthy fat, with non-starchy, low GI carbs. Don't eat processed or refined food. Eat real food. Stop counting calories and fat grams, instead, limit your carb/sugar intake. Cut out sugar, HFCS, artificial sweeteners, fruit juice, sodas, diet or otherwise. Avoid caffeine, nicotine, ephedrine, and all other stimulants. Avoid alcohol, as it will quickly sabotage your efforts.

As for skipping meals, what if I don't have time for breakfast?
Breakfast is the first meal of the day, no matter what time you choose to eat it. If you want your body and mind to perform at their best, you must provide them with the proper, most *efficient* fuel. Eat healthy meals. Please consider intermittent fasting. If you eat dinner, it

should be light with fat and protein only, no later than 5p. If you eat three meals, eat breakfast like a KING, lunch like a QUEEN, dinner like a PAUPER.

Eat clean. Eat *real* food.

What is the most effective way to safely increase my metabolism?

The safest, most effective way to increase your metabolism, thereby, lose weight, is by eating clean, healthy food. Building lean muscle mass will also help you burn body fat far more effectively.

But how do I really know what I'm eating?

When you grocery shop, you must make a new habit of reading the nutrition and ingredient panels. However, you need to really understand what you're reading so you can make better food choices. Take an interest. Be concerned. Expect more from the food you buy. (For more details, please read chapter 33, "How to Read a Nutrition Facts Label.")

What about meal replacement shakes and bars?

Beware of the diet products and programs that consist of drinking only a shake or eating a bar as two of your main meals. All one has to do is read the nutrition (and ingredient) labels to realize these products are often loaded with sugar. They are not nutritionally sound and will perpetuate your sugar/carb carvings. Furthermore, does anyone really eat these meal replacement bars *in lieu* of a meal? Most often, not. They typically eat them in addition to their regular meals, which equals way too many calories. If you were to only eat them as a primary meal, they would fall under the "low calorie dieting" category. While you may lose a few pounds by forfeiting a real meal for a meal replacement bar or drink, especially if you forfeited two meals, the pounds lost will be water weight and will occur only because you drastically cut back your caloric intake to bare minimum. This is low calorie dieting at its worst. You'll lose weight at first, as your glycogen stores are depleted, but then you'll plateau. At that point, your body will go into a starvation mode. This stage, if allowed to go too long, can be very dangerous. This is not a healthy way to lose weight, nor will you be able to keep the weight off lifelong.

How about a certain cereal that claims I can lose up to 6 pounds in 2 weeks?

Ahhh, operative words: *up to*. Nevertheless, this is merely another manipulative advertising blitz that will only fuel our obesity rate. Beware of this marketing ploy. For those who are not familiar, Kellogg's, the makers of Special K breakfast cereal, have been running a clever advertising campaign that claims you can, "Lose up to 6 pounds in 2 weeks!" *Reeeeally?* Pray tell. They claim it's possible by merely replacing two of your main meals by eating two bowls of Special K, along with 2/3 cup of skim milk, plus fruit. They also recommend you eat your third meal (and beverages) as you normally would, along with choosing snacks from fresh fruit, veggies, or one of their very own breakfast bars. Oh, how convenient.

Sorry to say, but this is another instance of incredibly poor nutritional advice, and, at the very least, it's misleading marketing. I was further taken aback when I read the list of ingredients: Sugar is third, and HFCS is fifth. Sugar is expected, *but HFCS in a breakfast cereal?* They can't be serious? Even I am stunned to see where they hide this sweetener. Post's Raisin Bran cereal is not much better. They claim you can "Lose 10 pounds" in pretty much the exact same manner. Their 4th ingredient is sugar, with corn syrup being fifth.

Kellogg's has since stopped running that particular ad, but I'd like to know why the FDA and FTC allow this type of deceptive advertising to go on for so long. They know damn well this is nothing but self-serving advertising, not to mention an unhealthy way to lose weight. Based on what you've learned here, would you care to tell me why these proposed diet plans wouldn't work?

Is it because they're basically low calorie with way too many high GI carbs?
Exactly. I'm so proud of you! It's not only low cal with nothing but high GI carbs (the cereal itself with the added sugar and HFCS, plus the skim milk and fruit), but Kellogg's also recommends you eat "normally" for your third meal, along with *whatever* beverages you want. Whoa! Knowing how most Americans eat and drink, that is most certainly asking for trouble. On top of being low calorie, this diet of high GI carbs will spike your insulin and deplete serotonin, perpetuating cravings, water gain, mood swings, all the many things that come from low serotonin. But, hey, most consumers won't care, because they will feel great while they're on this cereal diet since cereal is a very common comfort food. Just remember, that feeling of emotional comfort is only temporary.

And I suppose if I were to lose some weight, it wouldn't last. Right?
Yes, more than likely, you'll lose a couple of pounds. But it will only be temporarily, as this weight loss is false at best, and due only because you'll be consuming a lot fewer calories. With each "cereal meal" containing as little as 200 calories, including the skim milk and fruit, this is extremely low calorie. The little weight you lose will be from water and muscle, NOT body fat. The bigger problem is that when you start to eat normally again, you'll gain the weight back, plus 5–10% more. This type of dieting and highly questionable marketing practices has been, and still is, contributing greatly to our obesity epidemic. You must remember: DIETS DON'T WORK.

It's obvious very few give a damn about the consumer. It seems most only care about selling their product. No wonder we're getting so fat! Nothin' but lies!
This low calorie dieting is certainly old school thinking. But it serves the manufacturers quite nicely in their product promotion. With this type of marketing allowed, it's no wonder people no longer know what to eat. It's no wonder they're fed up. It's no wonder Americans are getting heavier by the minute. This is precisely why I wrote my books: To educate you, to help you make sense of it all. (Be sure to read my next chapter, "Marketing Scams That Are Making Us Fatter Than Ever!") **UPDATE:** The 100-Calorie Snack Packs, created by Kraft, have finally fallen short in sales. While they may be low in calories, they

are processed junk food—and oh so very addictive. Another shameful marketing ploy.

I will definitely read it. Now, if I shouldn't drink sodas, what can I drink?
Drink plenty of water and on a consistent basis. Here are several reasons why: About 60-70% of the body is water. The body's water supply is involved in almost every bodily function, including absorption, circulation, digestion, and excretion. Water is the key transporter of nutrients throughout the body. Water is vital for the proper functioning of the body and mental well-being. You need enough water to grow muscle. Water is a natural appetite suppressant and it hydrates your skin. Water is needed to help flush metabolized fat out of the body and regulate body temperature. When you think you're hungry, more often than not, you're just thirsty. Drink water <u>before</u> you get thirsty. Over 75% of all people are constantly dehydrated. A quick breakdown: 2% dehydration = thirst. 4% = dry mouth. 10% = heat stroke and even death.

Water, at room temperature, is one the best sources of hydration. However, your body also needs electrolytes, i.e., sodium, calcium, zinc, potassium, chloride, phosphate, and magnesium. These electrolytes must be replaced to keep the electrolyte concentrations within the body constant. (I use LyteShow.)

<u>Bottled Water Alert:</u> Bottled water is a 15-billion-dollar-a-year industry. Unfortunately, just as with countless other markets, the water industry has its share of less than honorable companies selling their goods. This market is not regulated. Recent studies show that over 31% of the 52 brands tested were contaminated with bacteria. The low-grade plastic that's used is also of serious concern, as it can easily leach toxins such as carcinogens and methyl chloride into the water, and, thus, the consumer. I urge you to please consider buying a quality distiller for your home or a simple water filter. You can then be guaranteed a much cleaner, healthier water. Plus, it will save you a ton of money over the years, greatly reduce the senseless trash, help save the lives of those who live near the plants that make the plastic bottles and cut deep into the profits made by Pepsi, Coca-Cola, and Nestle.

What do you do for quality water?
For home use, I filter my water always. To ensure I drink enough water throughout the day, I use a 64 oz, BPA-free, stainless steel container. Easier to track. I drink 50-60% of my body weight. I also drink it at room temp with lemon and electrolytes.

I like both of those ideas. That particular bottle, will help me keep track of how much I drink. But don't you agree that water gets rather boring?
Sometimes. But this is why I recommend my clients take quality water and squeeze in a touch of fresh fruit: grapefruit, strawberry, lemon, lime, etc. Adding sliced cucumbers can also be refreshing. Beware of bottled water that claims it's sugar free, as they're most often artificially sweetened with aspartame or sucralose/Splenda. Again, if something is sweet, you need to ask *why*. Read the ingredient panel carefully. Avoid carbonated/sparkling water due to the CO2 gas. They can cause bloating, IBS, weight gain, etc.

If I should avoid coffee, what then?

If you are truly healthy, which means at the very least, your serotonin is properly maintained, you should not have any desire for caffeine, coffee or otherwise. And, in lieu of drinking decaf coffee, consider caffeine free herbal tea, hot or cold. They come in so many different delicious flavors and with amazing health benefits.

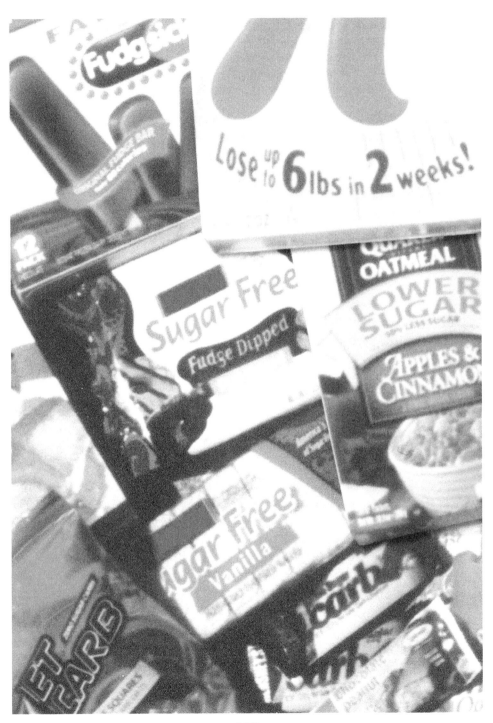

22

MARKETING SCAMS THAT ARE MAKING US FATTER & SICKER THAN EVER

What marketing scams are you talking about?
By far the worst and most despicable marketing scam perpetrated by the food industry is the harsh reality that all processed/junk food is intentionally poisoned by the food manufacturers. They add assorted harmful chemicals, chemicals that the FDA and FTC don't require to be accounted for on the food labels.

Harmful chemicals? **Why would they do this?**
The purpose behind the deliberate and precise manufacturing of this food is multi-dimensional. First, it's to get us addicted. *Why?* To keep us buying their products. Their next intention is to get us fat—and sick. *Why?* To enrich the medical and pharmaceutical industries. These chemicals, though, are not the only culprits here. The exorbitant amounts of sugar, HFCS, aspartame, MSG, etc., that are also added to this food, will equally cause addiction, obesity, depression, heart disease, and many other serious health issues.

This is all dreadfully alarming! It seems the food companies make us sick with their poisoned food, while the drug companies make us even sicker with their drugs! I'm finally starting to see the bigger picture here. It really is all about greed and with no regard for the consumer's health or well-being.
It is hard to accept that it truly comes down to corporate greed, which equals profits, huge profits. All the more reason to avoid processed, refined, canned, fast food, etc., and eat only real food as often as possible.

Are there other marketing scams I should beware of?
Oooooh, too many to mention. They're endless. Beyond the ruthless reality of what the processed food industry is really about, all one has to do is walk down any grocery store aisle and see just how many scams are intentionally put over on the consumer every day. I can't believe there are still so many fat free/low fat products on store shelves. In case you're not aware of this, while most snack food isn't generally a healthy choice, it's NOT the fat in the food that is making us fat. It is, however, the highly refined and processed, high GI carbs that this food is "made from" that is making us fat—and depressed. And, as I stated earlier, this food may not have fat, but they are LOADED with all types of sugar. If they're not jammed with sugar, they contain olestra, an indigestible fat substitute that has over 15,000 complaints, due to side effects ranging from gas, diarrhea, bloody stools, to cramps so severe that people had to be rushed to the ER. Once again, please avoid any

and all fat free/low fat food. (If the food has fat, watch out for trans fats.)

How awful! I hate to ask what's next?

After the terribly unsuccessful low fat movement promoted by the FDA and AMA, the next marketing scam launched by the food manufacturers (and eagerly allowed by the FDA, AMA, and FTC) was the low carb movement, followed swiftly by the net carb/impact carb campaign. Trust me, this is a *multi-billion-dollar marketing blitz* that will frighteningly exacerbate our current rate of obesity. At the same time, it will make those involved even richer.

With the FDA and FTC finally cracking down on more accurate labeling claims, I believe this whole net/impact carbs scheme resulted from this. This is nothing more than another pathetic marketing scam to confuse the unsuspecting and ever-trusting consumer. Just as the fat free/low fat food gave millions of consumers a free ticket to eat this food in abundance, so will this marketing tactic. The manufacturers would love you to believe this is "carb-friendly" food. All one has to do is read the label to realize this is not true. While some carbs do indeed breakdown more slowly, affecting blood sugar levels less dramatically, a carb...is a carb...is a carb. At the end of the day, all that matters is how many carbs you've consumed. And, are you active enough to burn up all those carbs?

Moreover, with deception running rampant in marketing and elsewhere, I would never believe any of these claims. It's nothing but a ploy. You need to read the label carefully. First and foremost, read the list of ingredients. This will give you a much better idea of what is actually in the product. Then count all carbohydrates, not just their claims of professed net carbs/impact carbs. Then determine whether or not you want to eat this type of product, and if you can afford to eat it. This is not free food. (Note: Warning letters were finally sent to food manufacturers indicating that the phrase "low carb" is not an FDA authorized term and should not be used.)

Then why is it on most carb products?

Good question, considering it's been used for several years. I think this is another reason why wannabe-carb-friendly food manufacturers transitioned their labels to claim "net carbs/impact carbs."

Why is all this marketing deception allowed?

It's allowed because the food industry is not properly regulated by the FDA or FTC. I also believe that it's another example of big business at work. The sugar industry, no matter what form it takes, is ENORMOUS. A lot of people make an extraordinary amount of money from these transactions. It is, again, only about profits. Another area to watch out for is the recent candy/chocolate industry packaging their many assorted sweets with "sugar free" labels. You must be wondering *why* something so deliciously sweet can be sugar free, aren't you? Well, if you haven't, it's time to start. Remember, if something is sweet, ask why. Those labels proudly screaming sugar free are not quite accurate. Those products contain a sweetener called maltitol. Because this particular type of sweetener supposedly has a minimal effect on blood sugar levels, the FDA does not consider it a sugar. Consequently, food manufacturers are allowed to make this claim.

How will I know what makes this food sweet?

I want you to first read the label to see how many sugar alcohols and "other carbs" the product is claiming. Please understand that these are simply an attempt to disguise the sugar. Trust me, nothing that sweet is ever sugar free, or good for you. Next, look in the ingredient section. This is where you'll find what actually sweetens the product.

What is maltitol?

Maltitol is an alternative sweetener known as sugar alcohols. There are those who claim it's a healthy choice for people with diabetes, because it has so little effect on blood glucose and insulin levels. But I, along with many others, disagree. Even if that claim were true, if you plan on indulging yourself with these wannabe sugar free sweets, you might want to have a diaper close by. This goes

for all sugar alcohols.

A what? *A diaper?* What are you talking about?

Maltitol, as with other sugar alcohols, are known for causing bloating, gas, and diarrhea. Ooooh! And, the pain can be quite bad. From my personal experience, although I didn't feel the typical sugar buzz after eating one of these sugar free bars that are loaded with maltitol, it did, though, make me crave more of the same. Worst of all, my stomach cramped painfully for hours soon after. It played such extreme havoc on my tummy that I refused to even throw this food down the hill, fearing I'd hurt the unsuspecting little animals that might eat it. This time, I threw them in the trash.

I can't begin to tell you how sorry I feel for most consumers, with all that the food manufacturers relentlessly throw at them. I'm sure the intentions of most people are to eat healthy, with an occasional treat. Yet with this type of marketing deception allowed, it's no damn wonder the poor consumer is getting fatter and fatter, even though they're eating nothing but the recommended fat free, sugar free, and carb free food.

I agree. I'm hoping you can help me make better sense of all of this. What else do I need to watch out for?

If I could walk down any given grocery store aisle with you, I'd show you literally hundreds of similar marketing scams. I'd have to say, however, that the protein and nutrition bars are one of the next biggest scams perpetrated on the consumer. *Why?* Because long before these bars became so popular, the only people who were eating them were athletes, people who really cared about what they put in their bodies, people who required extra protein. Now these bars are nothing but glorified, over-priced candy bars.

Oh, no, protein bars? Are you serious? I thought they were so healthy!

This is what the manufacturers would love for you to believe. These are nothing more than a highly processed food. Are you aware that most of these bars are loaded with sugar, often hidden under several different names other than "sugar?" (Not to mention most health bars are equally high in calories and hydrogenated oils.)

A different name from sugar? Such as?
Those names can range from glycerine, HFCS, corn syrup, fructose, molasses, honey, maltitol, xylitol, erythritol, etc. Some have over 25g of sugar in a 2 oz bar.

What if the bar claims it's sugar free?
First, I would highly doubt that claim. Then I'd read the label more closely and look for artificial sweeteners such as aspartame, erythritol, Splenda/sucralose, maltitol, xylitol, neotame, acesulfame-K, etc. You do not want to eat these. Next, you need to remember that whatever the amount of carbs in the bar, *and they are usually exorbitant amounts*, they will breakdown into sugar once consumed. You realize by now what sugar does to insulin levels and how it causes the body to crave more sugar, store fat, etc. Considering how competitive this market is, you need to do more than just read the nutrition labels. Their alleged claims of the amount of sugars within do not distinguish between refined and naturally occurring sugars. You have to read the ingredient panel to get more accurate information. The FDA requires all ingredients be listed in order of the quantity used.

Which sugars should I watch for?
All of them. Once again, those sugars can range from glycerin, high-fructose corn syrup, corn syrup, fructose, chocolate, to brown rice syrup, sucrose, maltodextrin, dextrose, maltitol syrup, cane sugar, xylitol, erythritol, chocolate liquor, etc. (Chapter 12, "The Many Faces of Sugar," lists many of the names under which sugar is disguised.)

Still doubting me? Okay. But please read on: Due to the extremely lucrative ($1.5 billion a year) yet fiercely competitive market, an independent lab revealed that many of the largest protein and health bar manufacturers were caught lying about the actual ingredients in their products. Out of 30 bars tested, an astounding 60% failed to meet their labeling claims. Only 12 bars passed on all criteria.

Are you serious? What were they lying about?
Although they lied about amounts of protein, the most prevalent problem, as well as the most disturbing to me, as a relatively trusting consumer, was not declaring total amounts of carbs. I'm not talking about small indiscernible amounts. I was shocked to see that half of all the bars tested exceeded their claimed carbs often by staggering amounts. One bar that claimed to be "low carb" with only 2g of carbs actually had 22g of carbs.

This can't be!
Sorry. Yes, it can. And there's more, I'm afraid. Eight of the top-selling bars also exceeded their sugar claims. These protein/health bars on average exceeded their sugar claims by

a whopping 8g. That equals 2 tbsp of sugar. A Snickers bar with a 300% markup. As bad as this is, it is exactly why I focus on the claim of "total carbs" versus just the sugar claim. *Why?* Because all those carbs they're claiming will turn into sugar either way. Yes, some carbs may burn slower, but both simple and complex carbs are recognized as sugar by the body. While these companies should be honest, I also realize that this particular industry can only survive if it's somehow able to disguise the sugar within.

Caught lying!

This is horrendous! No wonder I'm always craving a lousy protein bar. They're nothing but sugar! This also keeps me from losing weight. This should be illegal.
You're right. This is unacceptable. I find this type of marketing deception unconscionable. Those behind this deceit should be thrown in jail. Instead, the FDA simply comes in, warns them, possibly fines them, tells them to make the appropriate changes, and then allows them to continue doing business. It's one thing to make an honest mistake; it is entirely another matter to *knowingly* deceive the buying public, especially when it concerns things we are putting into our bodies. Don't believe for one second that these companies are innocent. They know all the tricks when it comes to getting consumers addicted to their products. Once addicted, we are their lifelong customer. No questions asked. So you see, a fine is merely a small part of the marketing game. (Of course, I know that throwing these people in jail is not an option, but the harsh reality is that monetary punishment for these huge companies will not deter them from future marketing scams.)

If that isn't disturbing enough, back in or around 2001, Atkins Nutritionals was also found guilty of deceptive product labeling on their diet/nutrition bars. The FDA sent out warning letters to them and 16 other companies, informing them that "their bars were misbranded, adulterated, and in violation of the Federal Food, Drug and Cosmetic Act." In addition, in August 2001, Tim Bryson of Alabama filed a class action lawsuit against Atkins Nutritionals for "intentionally misleading with regard to the characterization of the actual number of carbohydrates." Bryson's group won, with a settlement of $100,000. Now I have to ask: If we can't believe the company and/or the man who was the biggest advocate for low carb eating, *whom can we believe?* The protein bar market is a $7 billion market, with Atkins Nutritionals alone having sold more than $40 million worth of bars in the past year. Sadly, it always comes down to profits. Again, buyer beware. I tell my clients they need to look at protein bars, as nothing more than an expensive candy bar. In fact, I suggest that if they desire this kind of occasional treat, I'd rather have them eat a PayDay candy bar.

A PayDay? **You must be joking!**
No, not really. For starters, at least with a PayDay you'll know exactly what you're eating. There's no reason for the manufacturer to lie. It is what it is. Plus, all those peanuts will help lower the GI, as they're a good source of fat and high in protein. Funny, I've actually compared a PayDay's nutrition panel to several of the leading protein bars, and the PayDay is often a healthier choice. Personally, I have boycotted protein bars. Not only are

they not real food, but their manufacturers have cheated us, lied to us, and all with the greedy intention to get us addicted to their glorified candy bars.

Here's a great example of why you need to listen to your body: I woke up one night and thought to myself, "Hmm, a protein bar sure sounds good! *Excuse me? A protein bar?!* It's one o'clock in the morning! Why am I craving a protein bar?" This craving stunned me, particularly because the bars I was eating claimed a mere 2g of carbs/zero sugar. I hurried into my kitchen to read the label. Though, it of course, claimed only 2g carbs, I knew right then and there these bars were <u>not</u> what they pretended to be. I knew my mind was making me crave this bar for one reason only: SUGAR. It was only a few short months later that I read that all-telling article describing the extent of the deception found in the protein bar industry.

Sugar addiction—like any other DRUG habit.

Why do these companies lie to us and cheat us?
Profits. Huge profits. Don't be fooled, either. These companies know exactly what they're doing. So what if they have to pay a $10,000, $100,000, or even $1,000,000 fine. When you're making tens of millions, this is what these conglomerates call CDB (Cost of Doing Business). In the meantime, their deception is cleverly getting us <u>addicted</u>.

Most consumers buy a protein bar (or any product) that they see heavily advertised. They generally don't even bother to read the nutrition panel. They often blindly trust what the ads and packaging claim. Even if some take the initiative to read the nutrition facts to make sure these bars are a healthy choice, they won't read them time and time again. So if the consumer's favorite bar happened to be one of those caught lying, and, subsequently, had to start claiming the much higher amounts of carbs/sugar, this trusting consumer would never know this. This is, because, by then, this consumer is long addicted to these sugar-laden bars and will continue to keep buying them with the greatest of confidence.

Addicted?
Yes. <u>Sugar</u> is <u>ADDICTIVE</u>. The more bars we eat, the more bars we will crave. *Don't believe me?* I knew a man who used to have a $300-a-month protein bar habit. And trust me, this sugar addiction is like any other drug habit.

Food for thought: I feel it is important to include the first few and most crucial ingredients found in two very popular protein bars. The first is PowerBar. I selected this particular bar because it was the forerunner of this booming industry. All the more reason why I was so shocked to read its ingredients. I chose to feature Slim-Fast, as it's the bar that most women gravitate toward, because of the multi-million-dollar advertising campaign Slim-Fast runs each year to promote their weight-loss products. I was equally shocked.

<u>PowerBar/Original/Cookies & Cream Flavor</u>:

Ingredients: High Fructose Corn Syrup with Grape and Pear Juice Concentrate, Oat Bran, Maltodextrin, Milk Protein Isolate, Cookie Bits (Rice Flour, Sugar, Canola Oil, Alkalized Cocoa, Rice Starch, Sodium Bicarbonate, Salt), Brown Rice Flour, Almond Butter, Glycerin, etc.

I'm constantly amazed to see what food manufacturers put into our food, but I am further dismayed when it comes to supposedly healthy food choices such as protein bars. PowerBar's 1st ingredient is HFCS, the worst sugar there is. Plus, it has a staggering 45g of total carbs, 20g of which are sugar and 23g of "other carbs." After all that, it only has 9g of protein. Based on the primary ingredients, this is a candy bar, not a protein bar.

Slim-Fast Bar:

Ingredients: High-Fructose Corn Syrup, Milk Chocolate Flavored Coating (Sugar, Partially Hydrogenated Palm Kernel, Palm Oils, Partially Defatted Peanut Flour, Graham Cracker Cookie Pieces, Cocoa Processed with Alkali, Nonfat Milk Whey, Soy Lecithin, Salt, Artificial Flavor), High Maltose Corn Syrup, Soy Protein Isolate, etc.

I was stunned to see HFCS and corn syrup in Slim-Fast's various bars (and their other products). HFCS is also their 1st ingredient, followed by nothing but more sugar and hydrogenated oils. And whey, which is the actual protein, is the 10th ingredient.

So the real question is: Do these bars sound like real food, let alone healthy? I think not. My final warning: The better a bar tastes, the more sugar it will contain—and the worse it is for you.

How do you suggest I get my protein?

In lieu of these processed protein sources, please find a healthier source. Get your daily protein from real food, such as organic chicken, eggs, cod liver, duck, lamb, beef liver, turkey, fresh cheese, salmon, catfish, mahi-mahi, and shellfish. But first, please read the following chapter with an open mind for far healthier, kinder, and cruelty-free suggestions. While I sincerely appreciate this is a very sensitive and personal subject, I hope you will at least be willing to consider other options.

UPDATE: Weight Watchers 100% Whole Wheat Bread; another example of the power of branding. WW would love for you to believe their bread is healthy, and it will keep you thin. Sorry, not possible. First of all, it's a starchy carb. Secondly, the 2nd ingredient is gluten, 3rd is HFCS, followed by molasses, soybean oil, calcium propionate, mono and diglycerides, sodium stearoyl lactylate, datem, etc. Besides the sugar and assorted chemicals, this bread is definitely a high GI carb, one that will breakdown instantly into blood sugar. Therefore, their misleading carb count of 17g with just 2g of sugar actually = *17g of sugar,* based on this type of carb—and its harmful ingredients. Consumer beware. This type of deceptive food labeling is everywhere.

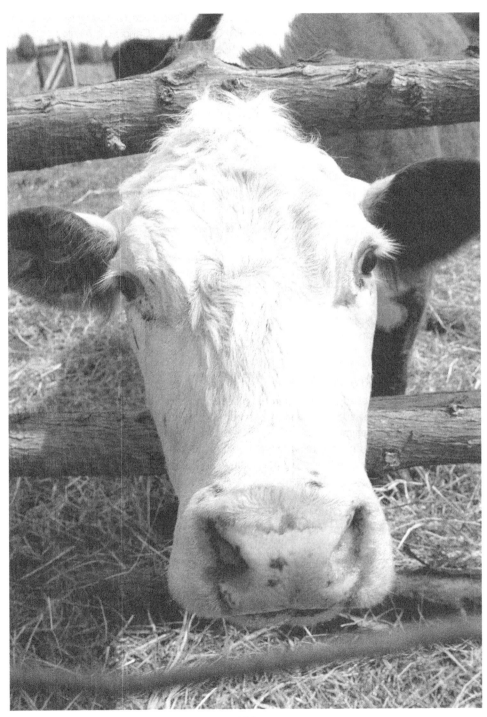

23

FROM PETTING ZOO TO DINNER TABLE
When did it go so terribly wrong?

Remember when our parents would eagerly take us to the petting zoo? As children, we were so amazed by these wonderful, loving creatures. We would feed them their favorite treats, reaching out with hope to simply touch them, feel their soft fur, to rub their pink little bellies. And ooooh my, if the little lamb or calf licked us, we would scream with such absolute delight! Ah, the pure joy of petting these many beautiful animals was *sooo exciting!* And this is why I <u>must</u> ask: *When did it go so terribly wrong? When did we go from wanting to love, adore, and care for these innocent animals to EATING THEM? How did it ever become acceptable to serve these animals at our dinner table?*

While I certainly respect the fact that we are each entitled to our own choices, I feel the desperate need to convey my very personal thoughts, concerns, and torment: Are you aware that more than **70 BILLION** of these once-cherished animals are slaughtered every year in the U.S. for food? Raising animals on factory farms is not only devastating to the land and to Mother Earth, but eating animals (especially red meat), is also bad for our health, leading directly to many diseases, including heart disease, heart attacks, strokes, diabetes, cancer, and obesity. The astronomical amount of food it takes to raise these millions of farm animals every year could, instead, be put toward ending world hunger. Don't forget that factory farming is responsible for *unfathomable* cruelty and senseless suffering for the animals involved.

First of all, would you eat your dog? Your cat? Your horse? Of course not. So, why do people eat pigs, which are known to be smarter than dogs, and equally as affectionate? Why do people eat cows, which are nothing but gentle, timid creatures? How could anyone *ever* eat a calf? The calf's only crime in life is to have been born a male. Hence, the severely short and tortured life of a veal calf. The same goes for every other animal, fowl, fish, etc., that we serve on our plates. All innocent creatures. Therefore, who gave us the right to end their lives, simply for our dining pleasure?

Shameful confession...

Personally, for over twenty years I had chosen not to eat most meat. Even though I felt I was doing my best for the rights of these animals, for my health, and Mother Earth, I am ashamed to say I continued to eat, somewhat guilt-free, chicken and turkey. Maybe because I was brought up in the Midwest, where the privately owned, small family farms were run dramatically different from the factory farms I speak of here, but I genuinely wasn't aware of any problems with eating eggs, butter, and cheese, as no animal was killed in this process. I recognized chickens and turkeys gave their life for me to enjoy their flesh, but it somehow seemed less tragic to eat them than it was to eat a cow, pig, or helpless little calf. I also thought these animals were at least treated humanely until the time of their death. Hence, I made it okay to eat them. However, I am now tormented by this—and dreadfully ashamed.

Why are you tormented?
Recently, I met Paul. Through our brief encounter, we discovered we were on the same path regarding health. He recommended I read *The Food Revolution* by John Robbins, heir to the "Baskin and Robbins" fortune. He told me it would be one of the most enlightening, and equally disturbing, books I would ever read. Oh, how right he was.

Now, I've long been aware of the horrific life veal calves live, as well as pigs and cows. But never was I aware of how chickens and turkeys are tormented in life—and at death. Based on what I read in Robbins' book, and then doing some additional research, I am repulsed and infuriated by what these animals, and all other farm animals, are forced to endure at the hands of "MANKIND." Moreover, our government doesn't do a damn thing to stop this cruelty. *But why is this allowed?* Cruelty is cruelty. Right? Be it to dogs, cats, children, or the elderly, there are laws to prevent such atrocities. Then please tell me why there aren't laws to protect innocent farm animals, as well?

I feel a frantic need to confess that I was shamefully ignorant when it concerned what farm animals go through in their short, tormented lives. I guess I wanted to believe these animals were at least treated humanely until the time of their death. *But this is not so.* The torture of these helpless animals is truly beyond words. For those who may not care about how these animals are treated, you should then, at the very least, be concerned about what these farm animals are forced to eat. *And why should this concern you?* Because what these animals eat is then eaten by you, when you eat them. The ultimate food chain. The ole' adage, "You are what you eat" was never more true.

What are you saying?
I'm saying that in addition to the many assorted hormones, antibiotics, drugs, etc., that these farm animals are fed to simply keep them alive in otherwise deadly conditions, to make them grow faster, produce more babies, eggs, milk, and so forth, their feed also contains everything from downed, diseased, cancerous, unwanted farm animals, to euthanized pets (yes, our beloved pets) to road-kill, along with every unimaginable animal part. This declared feed, which is commonly fed to farm animals, is considered an *acceptable* food source by our government.

You've got to be kidding me!
No, but I wish I were. I've long known that 99% of all commercial dog food is made from

this repulsive by-product, but I wasn't aware that the spread of such practice was so commonplace in the farming of animals that go to the marketplace, that marketplace being our dinner table. Then we wonder why so many people (and our pets) are getting cancer and other life-threatening diseases? So you see, there are many other concerns here beyond just the cruelty to these farm animals. If we eat them, we are, in essence, eating our own pets and all the other animals that were too sick to be properly slaughtered and sent to market. We are eating everything these animals were fed. I don't know about you but, it makes me ill just thinking about it.

Our government knowingly and willingly allows this horrendous abuse to go on, and they allow this feed to be fed to the farm animals. They also allow animals that are too sick, too damn ill to even walk to the transport truck, to be sold at auction, where these poor helpless animals are then again dragged, hauled, kicked onto the trucks in any way possible to get them to the actual slaughterhouse. If they survive that final ride, these animals are then further brutalized, all while they scream in such absolute terror, trying to run, desperate to get away, but they are too weak, too sick. The next time you'll see these helpless, diseased animals will be at your local grocery store, wrapped in cellophane, sold under desensitized names: "Bacon. Ham. Sausage links. Babyback ribs. Hot dogs. Hamburger. Steak. Prime rib. Headcheese. Sweetbread. Saltimbocca. Lamb chops."

This can't possibly be true! How could anyone allow this to go on?
Well, it is true. It is literally HELL ON EARTH for these helpless animals. In addition to refusing to eat cow or pig, and never ever eating veal, knowing now how chickens and turkeys are treated, how they're caged, driven insane, forced to cannibalism, self-mutilation, and worst of all, how they're so brutally killed, I can't possibly keep eating them. These animals were not put here for us to eat them, more so TORTURE them. As for most dairy products, unfortunately, by eating them I support the violence and slaughter of milking cows, and *indirectly*—the veal industry. Therefore, I must find healthier, much kinder substitutes for any products made from cow's milk.

I'm more than eager to rethink my diet, but my husband loves his steak!
Yes, most men love meat. Nevertheless, I plead with you to at least watch "Meet Your Meat," an exceedingly disturbing video narrated by Alex Baldwin. Download it for free at meetyourmeat.com. Watch it alone, with your husband, or grab a friend. You will be positively mortified by what you see. The images still haunt me months later. Then go to PETA.com (People for the Ethical Treatment of Animals) and veganoutreach.org. Each of these Web sites will show you just exactly what these farm animals go through in their far too short and tortured lives and at their death. Also, consider reading John Robbins' book. You owe it to yourself to open your eyes to the numerous health risks involved—*and the unthinkable cruelty.*

I thought you said eggs were good for us?
They are. This is why I must respectfully disagree with vegetarians who claim eggs, butter,

and cheese are unhealthy due to their fat/cholesterol content. Sorry, but this is another example of old school nutrition. The body and brain thrives on healthy fat. Although I will try to get my needed fat from olives, assorted oils, nuts, and avocados, I still believe eggs are crucial to good health, as they are a perfect protein, a perfect food. If I could get my eggs fresh from a local farmer, knowing the laying hens had been fed properly and had not been subjected to abuse, I would most definitely keep eating eggs. To reiterate, we to need to eat dietary cholesterol to shut down our internal production of same. Therefore, as I begin this new journey, I have to admit I'm struggling a bit about how to make sure I give my body all that it needs without contributing any further to the carnage of these innocent animals.

What about those who say these animals are raised precisely for food?
It's one thing to raise animals for food because we have no other options, but we do have options. To ignore those options, only to make these animals suffer throughout their entire young lives, to then be skinned and/or boiled alive, or dismembered while they're still conscious, is beyond comprehension! I have to ask: *Who is the animal here?* Just because we're at the top of the food chain, just because we don't speak their language, just because we don't feel their pain, doesn't make it okay.

However, I am not about to force my beliefs (or agony) on anyone else. We each have freedom of choice. So if, and only after you and yours watch the video, you still insist on eating meat and dairy, then I highly recommend you buy organic, free-range, antibiotic-hormone-cruelty-free food. It may cost a bit more, but your health is at stake here. It's also about helping put an end to the senseless abuse these animals are made to endure. Buying this food will hopefully, in some way, help ensure that these animals are at least treated humanely, fed properly, and when the time comes, *killed with compassion*. (WARNING: The FDA doesn't currently have regulations on what "free range" really means. Free range animals are not necessarily free of exploitation. They certainly aren't running free, enjoying fresh air, or the feel of cool green grass on their little feet as the packaging wants us to believe. Beware of these claims.)

I unquestionably want to do the right thing for the health of my family, while not contributing to the senseless slaughter of farm animals. But how will I know if these animals were truly free range, without hormones or drugs—and treated humanely?
You won't, unfortunately, not until the FDA enacts stricter guidelines—and then actually enforces them. I can only suggest that you try to shop at stores that focus on healthier, farm-fresh, organically grown food. Whole Foods, Sprouts, Trader Joe's, Wild Oats, Mother's Market, and Farm-to-Market are all excellent stores to patronize.

As terribly disturbing as all of this is, I believe most people are wonderfully compassionate, with no desire to hurt another living thing. We could literally be driven to tears, though, if we focused on all such brutality and misfortune in the world. Obviously, it goes far beyond farm animals. I also realize that we each have to find our own way. I can only hope that we all do our very best to give of ourselves in whatever way we can to help others and to stop cruelty to both mankind and animals.

To conclude this highly emotional chapter: At least cut your meat and dairy intake back to half. If everyone did this, this alone could help stop the suffering of billions of animals. Also take a moment to write to Congress and demand laws that will protect farm animals. Boycott companies known for cruelty. Refuse to buy fur. Find a way to reach out beyond your own needs. Find a worthy cause. Donate. Don't turn your back. Speak up. Dare to defend others, both man and beast. And, please, at the very least, eat with a conscience.

WARNING: KFC is one of the worst when it comes to torturing animals. From slamming live birds against walls, stomping on them when they refuse to die, to boiling them alive. 850 million chickens are viciously slaughtered each year by KFC. **NEWS UPDATE:** KFC refused to implement kinder, more humane treatment for even one, single helpless bird! *Is this really so much to ask?* It's bad enough they give their life for us, but do they need to be tortured in the process? No. Boycott KFC. Butterball is also torturing their birds, even sexually. Please do not buy Butterball turkeys or any other bird. To witness Butterball's House of Horrors, go to goveg.com/feat/butterball/butterball.asp.

McDonald's, the largest purveyor of beef, was under fire for allowing, on average, one in every one hundred cows to go through the assembly line ALIVE. Which means these cows were skinned and dismembered while fully conscious! *Talk about horror!* I can't even begin to grasp the suffering involved here. PETA and other animal rights activists have fought for years to get McDonald's to address this serious issue. McDonald's finally made changes to ensure their cattle are killed humanely. With regard to their chickens, unlike KFC, both McDonald's and Denny's have taken critical steps toward implementing CAK (Controlled-Atmosphere Killing), the most humane method of slaughtering chickens. Tyson, PETCO, and Iams are also under fire for cruelty to animals. Boycott these and any other companies that use animals for testing or subject them to cruel and inhumane treatment.

NEWS UPDATE: California voters approved Proposition 2 by a large majority, which will ban some of the worst cruelty to animals who are raised for food in that state. Thrilling victory! Now, if only the rest of the states, and world, would follow.

The women below are just an example of the hundreds of clients I've worked with.
They are exceptional examples, though, of what is possible, if you follow my lead.

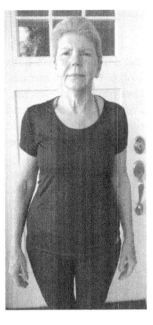

Age is nothing, but a number.
Age 66 & 67

Connie has achieved extraordinary
success with me.
Off wine. Off caffeine.
Off high GI carbs. Off deadly statin.
HDL 102. Trigs 48.
Osteopenia reversed.
Lean muscle mass & low
body fat with a 26" waist.
Feels fantastic! Looks incredible!
Inspires others!
She shares in our partnership
with such sincere
appreciation and respect for all
that I'm trying to do for her.
I am grateful.

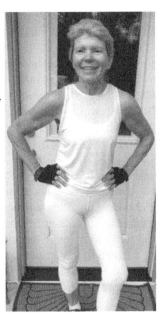

Fierce. Focused. Female.
Age 51 & 53

Cami, talk about motivated.
This woman refused to fail.
Off her wine and junk carbs.
Size 22 to an 8.
Trigs dropped 144 to 70.
HDL up 51 to 73.
She lost 11.5" off her waist,
10.5" off her insulin gauge,
10.75" off her hips,
75 lbs, and 13.8% body fat.
Yet Cami's success goes far
beyond her exceptional
physical transformation. She
made herself a priority above her
job, junk carbs, and wine.
Her whole outlook on life has
changed. Besides looking
incredible, her rewards are
innumerable! She shares in
our partnership with sincere
conviction and appreciation.
I am grateful.

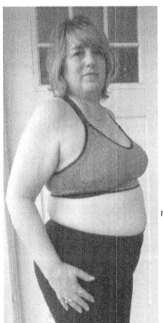

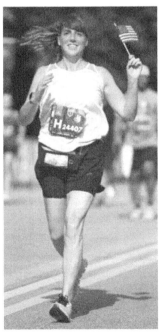

To view more transformations, please visit bodybyphoenix.com/weight-loss-transformation-video/

24

EXERCISE, NUTRITION & HORMONES
A tricky balance to achieve optimum health

Besides eliminating high GI carbs/sugar, processed food, and caffeine, what else do you recommend for this healthy lifestyle?
You must start some sort of exercise routine, even if it's just 30 minutes a day. (An hour for children.) Please don't tell me you don't have the time. Everyone has 30 minutes to devote to themselves. If you don't, you need to rethink your life. Some believe working out or having a trainer is a "luxury." It is not. If you want to be healthy and be around for your family, you must take care of *you.* God knows some women are never short on time when it comes to getting their nails, eyebrows and eyelashes done, shopping, or socializing over a decadent latte. Men, you always find the time to watch TV, golf, play video games, or hang with the fellas. So please, please, please, make the time to exercise. You will feel so much better about yourself—mentally, emotionally, and physically. There are few things in life that will return so much, as regular exercise.

What do you suggest?
There are so many things you can choose from. It can be as easy as playing ball with your children, going for a brisk walk with your dog, swimming some laps, riding your bike, surfing, skiing, dancing, playing golf, taking up yoga, or working in the garden. Maybe you're healthy enough to play tennis, handball, shoot hoops, kickbox, or lift weights. The key is: Do anything to get your body moving. Do it alone, with a friend, or with your spouse. Remember, competition is great for the soul. It motivates and inspires.

Why is exercise so important?
There are so many glorious benefits from exercising. For starters, exercise is a fantastic way to naturally stimulate the production of serotonin, norepinephrine, and endorphins, all of which help alleviate depression and mood swings, while improving sleep and libido. It suppresses your appetite and lowers your risk for heart disease, obesity, osteoarthritis, osteoporosis, diabetes, and other serious health conditions. Exercise slows the signs of aging, boosts growth hormone and metabolism, as well as strengthens the cardiovascular system. Exercise builds lean muscle and strong bones. The more lean muscle you have, the more calories/fat your body will burn, and it will burn them long after you've stopped exercising. I can't say this enough: The most effective way to maintain long-term fat loss, to achieve a lean, yet strong, healthy body with minimal fat is to build lean muscle mass. The right combination of a healthy diet and living a healthy lifestyle will further ensure your success. (The 5 will help you adhere to both.)

Weight training and a healthy diet are the best ways to get rid of cellulite. Stop wasting your time, money, and hopes on those expensive and most definitely useless creams that promise you leaner, smoother thighs and buttocks by simply slathering on their magic potions. They do not work. If you want to get rid of that lumpy and unsightly skin, *live a healthy lifestyle*. That means a diet that is devoid of sugar, alcohol, artificial sweeteners, damaged fats, refined and processed food. Focus on healthy fats, quality proteins, plenty of water, consistent exercise, and low GI carbs.

What do you do to stay in shape?
Though I played every sport growing up, weight training has long been my priority. I started weight training at 18. Working as a personal trainer at 19. I've tried different things along the way, but resistance training is what allows me to create the physique I want. It's the most effective, most efficient way to build lean muscle, strong bones, deplete fat stores, and actually sculpt my body. Weight training has proven to not only dramatically slow the signs of aging, but it has also been shown to *reverse* the aging process. (BTW: I train just as much for my mental state of mind, as I do for my physical body.)

How often do you train?
I'm fortunate to maintain my physique with two to three days of training a week, devoting just 40 minutes per session. Considering I've now been in and out of gyms for most of my life, I know exactly what I need to do. I know what works best for my body. I also push myself hard throughout each session. With very little rest, I get my heart rate up, as well. Now I know there are those who train 5, 6, or even 7 days a week, with 2 or 3 hours per session. No, thanks. I want a life outside the gym, just as I know you will, too. Also, most people overtrain. They don't realize that it's in the recovery period that they make gains. Don't get me wrong, though, I'd rather see people in the gym making an effort than not at all. The more intense type of training is rarely necessary, unless you're a professional athlete or competing. I just don't want this to discourage those who are starting out. Believe me, you will not have to spend every waking moment in the gym to get a strong, sleek, healthy, and attractive body. On the other hand, with so few days, you'll have to make sure your workouts are focused and consistent. You'll also have to commit to a healthy diet and lifestyle, if you sincerely hope to achieve your fitness/wellness goals. One will not work without the other. To ensure you eat this healthy diet, maintain your serotonin.

Do you still train others?
Yes, I actually opened, Body by Phoenix, a private weight loss, anti-aging, and personal training studio in Marietta, GA. I invite you to view my work at bodybyphoenix.com. You can watch my before/after video of my many amazing clients and see just how quickly, and dramatically, their bodies change. It is stunning to see. However, as I always tell my clients: "I am only as good, as they allow me to be. It is, after all, a partnership." I also consult and offer programs to those who live elsewhere.

How often do your clients train?

As a trainer with over 44 years of diverse expertise, I help my clients achieve remarkable results with just two days a week. And, only 30 minutes per session. (I condense an hour plus into 30 minutes.) I call it "time efficient training." With just two 30 minute sessions per week, we dramatically change their bodies. With hard work and perseverance on the floor, moreover, with their nutrition, we've mitigated various addictions, alleviated depression, anxiety, depression, and insomnia, reversed diabetes and hypertension, reduced harmful trigs, while significantly improving cholesterol panels, etc. At the same time, we sculpted firmer, more defined arms and buttocks; stronger, sexier backs and chests; shoulders that are strong and sculpted; smaller, sleeker waists; tighter abs; significant loss of body fat and much better overall body composition. On top of that, they also achieved much healthier mental/emotional attitudes. My role, as their trainer and nutritionist, is to teach, motivate, encourage—and to expect more from them, than they expect from themselves.

Denise, one of my clients from CA, told me she had some girlfriends who were raving about her new physique. Then, as some sadly will do, they tried to say her phenomenal shape was due solely to the fact that she could "afford a trainer." Denise quickly respond-ed, "What do you think, this comes easy, without any effort on my part? Hell, *this* (as she pointed to her body) takes HARD work! While I choose to have a trainer, my trainer is not the one doing the work! She's not the one doing the damn exercises. I am!" Denise was correct. It is the client who does the work. I am merely the driving force. I was proud of her for saying this, because no matter the client, their results are only as good as the amount of effort they're willing to put in on the floor and with their nutrition.

Far too many women are unhappy with their bodies, so one more story: Lisa, my client, was headed to the beach with her daughter and a few of her college buddies. As they wan-dered down the shore, Lisa noticed they were walking quite a ways behind her. Though she felt a bit left out, she thought maybe her daughter and the others were embarrassed to be seen with her. After all, she was "the mother" and 30 years older than they were. Only when she jokingly mentioned it later to her daughter did she find out the real reason. Lisa was told they were keeping their distance because "she looked so much better in a bikini than they did!" It was *they* who were embarrassed to be seen next to her. Lisa, being the humble woman that she is, was stunned by this admission. She was, nevertheless, flat-tered. Now, can you imagine that at 51 years of age, you could look better than a group of 20-year-olds and to do this in a BIKINI? Well, imagine it. Then believe it, because it's possible if you're willing to make the effort.

SOME OF MY GA CLIENTS: Please note, I only measure waist, insulin gauge (widest girth of stomach), and hips, along with body fat. In just 3 weeks, a client's body is changing, losing anywhere from 5-15". Jane, 50, in just 10 weeks lost 15.75". In 6 months, she lost an exceptional 25". In 13 months, she lost 46", 85 pounds, 9% body fat, and I reversed her osteopenia. What I loved even more is that when people told Jane how fabulous she looked, she humbly replied, "Thank you! And, I *feel* fabulous, too!"

Rhonda, 64, had never trained before, yet in just 7 weeks, her bloated tummy was gone. She was lean and so much stronger. In 9 months, and for the first time in her entire adult life, she was wearing a size 6. I dropped her trigs 119 points. HDL up by 36 points. Kim, I reversed her diabetes, weaned her off an antidepressant, caffeine, and nightly bottle of wine. Marla, 49, went from depressed, anxious, overweight, and drank too much, to now looking like a gymnast, a happy one at that. Nancy, 60, wanted me to keep her healthy enough to enjoy her grandkids. At 67, she was doing pushups with a grandchild on her back. At 70, she has one helluva right hook. Tina, 31, I weaned her off her caffeine, alcohol, and an antidepressant, alleviated her depression, anxiety, and cravings for crap carbs. She lost 5" off her insulin gauge in just 24 days. Her mental health transformation took me only 60 days. She's never felt better. Raechelle, 40, came to me frustrated that she looked four months pregnant. She lost 18" in 3.5 months. I alleviated her sugar cravings and insomnia. She's now down 26" and 6.5% body fat. Kathie, 60, lost 17" in five months and I weaned her off her antidepressant. Dr. Kathy, 54, overweight, depressed, ate crap, drank 3 glasses of wine nightly, with a pot of coffee every morning, lost 12.5" off her insulin gauge in just 6 months. Her trigs dropped 93 points, HDL up 33 points, and I weaned her off her antide-pressant in 60 days. Mary, 43, tired, overweight, drank, and ate poorly. She now inspires women everywhere. Jackie, 55, said she only needed a "little tweaking." Yet I took her from a size four to a zero in only 8 weeks, while taking 6" off her insulin gauge. Kristi, 51, came to me frustrated with a diet program she had been on, a diet that "insisted" every meal have fruit, and if not fruit, a serving of wine. *What?!* This had to be a joke! It wasn't. She was miserable and so hungry she ate a bottle of chewable vitamins. With me, and in only 90 days, she learned what was actually healthy to eat, lost 9" off her insulin gauge, 5" off her waist—and she never went hungry. She's now training for a triathlon.

Sherry, Pat, Sharon, Paula, Kim, Jennifer, Cami, Connie, Tiffany, LaShanda, Melinda, and so many other women who have trained at my Body by Phoenix studio, have also trans-formed their bodies and mental/emotional health. They're leaner! Feel better! Happier! Healthier! Self-confident. Off meds. Diabetes reversed. Trigs lowered. HDL higher. Look 10-20 years younger! No face-lift needed. They get so much more out of L-I-F-E. They, in turn, inspire so many others. This is what my work is about. (Please read testimonial page.)

Woooo! I'm inspired and further motivated. What are your personal goals?
My goals are simple: Remain physically strong, maintain muscle and bone mass, and mental capacity. Keep my body fat around 13-14%, trigs: 40ish, HDL 77+, BP stable, waist 26"—and all so I can reduce my risks for disease, and remain independent, as I age.

How do you maintain and define your muscle mass?
My routines vary, as I need muscle confusion. I train each muscle group directly twice a week. Nutrition plays a major role (80%) in my, and your, success. Maintenance is a lot easier than when you first begin training. It's like putting money in the bank: The more you invest in your health early on, the more you will get in return as the years go by. Take the challenge. There's no better time to start than right now.

Women, please **MAKE YOURSELF A PRIORITY**. It is not being selfish. We, as women, are the caregivers. You need to get, and/or remain healthy, for those you love and already take care of, be it the husband, boyfriend, kids, grandchildren, home, job, pets, parents, in-laws, etc. TAKE CARE OF YOU. So you can take care of them. Put down the lattes, get rid of the fake nails and eyelash extensions, weekend cocktails with girlfriends, Brazilian bikini wax, Starbucks, all those things that give you nothing in return. Invest that money in your health. Hire a proven trainer, and eat, as you've learned here. It will give you back a thousandfold. I promise!

As for you men, please do likewise. If you were to cut out your double espressos, beer, martinis, video games, and nights out with the boys, you, too, would have more than enough money to afford a trainer and/or gym membership.

You're right. It's all about priorities. I can cut out my sugary lattes and do my own waxing and nails. Now, how do you feel about jogging?
First of all, great attitude. Secondly, I don't recommend jogging for my clients, more so, long distance, and most definitely, not for my older female clients. There are many other wonderful ways to get your cardio rather than the harsh impact on your joints/organs that comes with jogging. Most gyms have elliptical trainers. They offer a smooth, non-impact, and effective cardio workout. You can also ride a stationary or street bike. Swimming is another great option. Or lace up and punch a heavy bag. Or...turn up the music and move.

Can I just do cardio and achieve good results?
No. Cardio is a muscle depleting exercise. If you want to sculpt your body, and burn more body fat, grab the weights. I watch so many people in the gym running endlessly on a treadmill. They run literally forever, and yet, over the months, sometimes years, I never see any difference in their bodies. Besides the fact that you must eat a healthy diet to see changes, you also need *resistance* on your muscles to "sculpt" them. In addition, having LBM is one of the best ways to burn body fat, as muscle is remarkably active—and 24 hours a day. Compare this to when you raise your metabolism through jogging; its fat burning benefits last only while you're doing it and a few hours after you're done. So, which sounds more effective to you? I know I want my body to work *with* me, not against me. Having LBM gives me numerous health benefits long after I leave the gym.

CARDIO ALERT: Many experts are now saying that the high level of stress that most cardio exercises have on your heart is too much. Thus, the stimulation brought on by intense cardio is actually breaking the body down, rather than building it up. Case in point: How many times do we hear about the athletic 45-year-old man dying of a heart attack, while he's out jogging? Once again, I've never done a regular, high impact cardio workout.

What would your perfect wellness program include?
It is mind, body, and spirit: That includes 8-9 hours of quality sleep, healthy food, two large meals, no dinner, 55% of my weight in water, three days a week weight training, and

walking daily with my beloved dogs. Massage and chiropractic care every six weeks. I also devote time to enrich my mind and spirit, be it simply laying quietly in the arms of my loving husband, enjoying my dogs and Mother Nature, rescuing animals in need, riding horses, music, photography, the beach, swimming, writing, and teaching myself Italian.

That all sounds wonderful. Now, how do you keep your stomach so flat?
I personally don't go for the chiseled ab look, rather, lean and flat, it's simple: Keep my serotonin levels balanced. This makes it so easy to control my eating habits. As I've said a dozen times, there is no effort whatsoever for me to eat healthy. I never feel cheated, deprived, or hungry. I'm sure this is completely the opposite of all the diets you've tried. Those diets not only left you hungry, but they also made you radically irritable. Who wouldn't be, when you're deprived of food? An added bonus of healthy serotonin levels is that while you're losing the weight, your mood will be better than ever. Those who have been gracious enough to notice my efforts (in particular, the women), assumed that I either did not eat or that I did a ton of ab work. I hated to disappoint them, but I told them I never go hungry, I never feel deprived, and I only train my abs directly twice a week. Furthermore, no one could ever do enough crunches to keep their waistline lean and without that typical little (or not so little) pooch if they don't eat healthy. I don't care how intense or how many ab exercises you do, diet is crucial to achieving a lean body with *minimal* body fat, which then greatly contributes to lean muscle definition, abs and otherwise. (Please read chapter 27, "GOT ABS?")

Didn't you say our stomach is our insulin gauge?
The stomach is what most accurately reflects one's eating habits. Go ahead. Measure yours. This is what you need to pay close attention to, because it's the most harmful weight we carry. Your waist is about one inch above your belly button. Your insulin gauge is the widest girth of your stomach, right at your belly button. It is the best indicator of how healthy you're eating, or not. My stomach is, hence, the first place I'll see the effects of eating poorly.

A perfect example of our waist being our insulin gauge is easy enough to observe if you look at the many girls and young women who wear the latest fashion: skin tight, low-riding pants. Sadly, for most of those who wear them, their little tummies bulge out, rolls of fat hang over, and then, on top of that, they wear a belly jewel, which draws even more attention to their pudgy and not so flattering waistline. Maybe this is indeed the style, but I can't believe these young ladies think this looks appealing. Do they not look in the mirror, to see how they look from all angles? Not only is this not attractive, but my primary concern is that these ladies are also so young and already headed for serious weight problems. For starters, their waistline reflects their risk of developing diabetes. It doesn't take a genius either to know *why* they're getting so heavy, so young. Rarely do I ever see one who doesn't have a large soda in hand with a bag of chips, happily munching away. As for the boys, they're hiding their excess weight under all those baggy, hip-hop clothes.

You just described my teenage daughter. All she eats is cereal, Hot Cheetos, bagels, and sodas! She's gained 15 pounds, moodier than ever, but no matter how much I try to help her, she refuses to listen. What can I do?

Take what you've learned here and put it to use. People need to realize that no matter one's age, low serotonin affects most of us in one way or another. Whether it's cravings, weight gain, mood swings, depression, rage, PMS, or ADD, I suggest you get your daughter on 5-HTP to help control both her cravings and mood swings. Plus, stop buying all those high GI carbs. Why tempt her? Also, try to get her motivated to start working out.

Are you saying healthy levels of serotonin will help control her angry outbursts?

Yes. One of the most common side effects of serotonin fluctuating drastically is fits of rage, emotional outbursts, and being quicker to anger. This comes from ingesting too much sugar, which then spikes your insulin, followed by your serotonin soaring, then plummeting. (The psychiatry industry would diagnosis it as mental illness—and either lock us up, or drug us until we surely lost our minds.) Most women, however, know that all-consuming feeling that suddenly comes from out of nowhere. We feel absolutely fine one moment, yet the very next second, we feel our head ever so slowly spin around. Our claws come out. Our seething words cut with precision, like that of a rusty, jagged knife. Our facial expressions alone, could kill. We are ready to literally rip the flesh off anything that moves. Most often it is our unsuspecting mate. We know our anger isn't warranted, but we can't stop it. As quickly as this angry-terribly-unattractive-outburst takes us over, it's gone. Whew! We take a deep sigh and quietly pray we will be ignored, more so *forgiven* for this irrational outburst. *But hold the laughter, gentlemen.* Before you dare judge us, you, too, are more than capable of these fits of psychotic rage. God knows I've dated more than a few men who are a perfect case study of this scenario. Nonetheless, man or woman, it's not a pretty sight. I at least know where this unjustified anger comes from.

Bioidentical hormone therapy versus deadly HRT

You are so right! Unfortunately, I witness this drastic mood shift not only in my daughter, but also myself and my husband. While men so unfairly accuse women of being premenstrual or simply a bitch, I often wonder what their excuse is.

Speaking of menstrual cycles, it's imperative that I comment on the many young women who allow their doctors to put them on the pill. If you're wondering why you feel so bloated, fat, and irritable, well, don't look any further. I know birth control is a very personal decision, but the pill comes with numerous health risks, from weight gain, stroke, to even death. Please consider another form of birth control. Then, when menopause comes knocking, please understand, ladies, that it is <u>not</u> a disease. Menopause is a natural stage of the aging process. It's perfectly natural to want to treat your symptoms, but beware of the pharmaceutical industry's proposed HRT (Hormone Replacement Therapy). These drugs have proved to be deadly. While the drug companies promised aging women far better health, the studies that came back proved to be extremely alarmingly. Women who were on HRTs were actually having more heart attacks, more heart disease, more strokes, more fatalities. At the very least, these women were heavier, more bloated than ever before. All you have to do is look around at most women over 50 to see the results of those purported wonder drugs.

But, please, is anyone *really* that surprised? I mean, after all, these drugs are not natural, they are synthetic. Premarin, produced by Pfizer, once a $3-billion-a year drug, contains over 50 horse estrogens from pregnant mares' urine. *Horse urine?* How could anyone have ever believed this would work in a woman's body? Horse urine is not only completely foreign to the female body, but the entire medical concept is also insane. As if that isn't frightening enough, the drug companies cruelly abuse these beautiful horses for years, slaughtering their foals immediately. Then, after they've served their purpose, the mares are also killed. Please, ladies, BOYCOTT THIS DRUG. Treatment for menopause should focus on treating your symptoms. Research your options. If you need estrogen replacement, use real hormones. Real hormones do *not* come from horse urine. I'm speaking about *natural bioidentical hormones* such as estradiol, estriol, estrone, DHEA, testosterone, and progesterone. Find a doctor and compound pharmacist who are trained in bioidentical hormone therapy.

I started getting migraines and hot flashes last year. My blood tests confirmed that, at 44, I was going into perimenopause. My doctor insisted I go on the pill to help balance my low levels of estrogen. In less than three weeks, I gained 10 pounds! It was all in my stomach, like a big fat water balloon.
If you gained this weight since the time you started taking the pill, then I'd say it's more than likely. This is why it's important to learn to think for yourself and do some research. Don't let your doctor put you on the pill, HRT, or any other med without weighing the countless risks. Here's where you'll definitely have to listen to your body. Hopefully, your doctor will run the appropriate tests, but finding the right balance with the various bi-hormones takes time and patience. Don't ignore your body when things don't feel right.

Are you taking them?
Yes. I was 42 when blood tests confirmed I was in perimenopause. I was shocked. Suddenly I felt old. Nonetheless, all my primary caregiver could offer me was HRT. No, thanks. I chose to endure the weekly migraines and occasional hot flash. By age 44, my migraines and hot flashes were far more frequent, along with joint pain, and I wasn't feeling as sexually motivated. I knew I had to do something. Thankfully by now, though, I had a new doctor, an ob/gyn who was offering hormones. Due to my symptoms, she, also, suggested a low dose of the pill. Considering even at 16 years of age I had refused to take the pill due to its many risks, I wasn't about to start. Bioidentical hormone were my only choice. Between her and my compound pharmacist, they designed a regimen consisting of testosterone, progesterone, estrogen, and DHEA. Finding the right dose for the test/DHEA was easy. The estrogen and progesterone proved to be a little more difficult. Considering my body type, i.e., tall, athletic, minimal body fat, and naturally small breasts, is the type that produces, and sustains, with very little estrogen.

Any change in estrogen is, therefore, felt immediately. I tried several forms, but each one came with side effects, side effects I was fortunate enough to tune into and tell my doctor about. She then quickly pulled me off of them.

What were the side effects?
I was first put on an estrogen pill. Within 10 days, I gained weight around my waistline, and my stomach was bloated. I suddenly felt fat as a pig. As all women know, feeling F-A-T will no doubt lead to frustration and bitchiness. I also felt a bit wired. I knew the only thing I had changed was adding the hormones. I decided to check my BP. Sure enough, it had gone from my average 100/60 to a much higher 165/75. Based on the research, I knew about 8% of women have this reaction to oral estrogen. I stopped taking it.

Though it does indeed take time and patience to find the combination that works best for your individual body, if your hormones have declined, they're certainly worth the effort. My goal is to help protect my female health, my heart, mind, body, and yes, my sexuality, via bi-hormones. But there must be a proper balance. This requires tuning into your body, listening to your body. Work closely with your doctor and compound pharmacist. Be sure they start you on them one at a time so you can monitor any possible side effects. Whatever you choose, please ladies, do NOT accept that awful-bloated-tummy-bitchy-dried-up-sleepless-always-tired-can't-remember-nothin'-lonely-lack-of-passion-sexual-desire, as normal. It is not. It does not have to be part of the aging process.

<u>UPDATE:</u> Most effective manner in which to test hormones levels is salvia, not blood. Most effective, safest way to take them is transdermal versus pills.

Anything would be better than the way I feel now. My mood has been horrendous, never mind the extra weight. What about my husband? Can he benefit from them?
Yes. After 40, men should be concerned with maintaining their hormones, primarily testosterone. A testosterone deficiency is exhibited by a diminished sexual drive and difficulty in getting and/or maintaining an erection. Lack of energy, loss of height, bone mass and muscle tissue, plus, being a bit more irritable, are also common. Not all men lose testosterone. Some men don't get depressed; they maintain strength, energy, and muscle mass, and remain sexually active until the day they die.

I have to be terribly honest and say it all sounds just too good to be true.
I know. But, just remember, the research I'm sharing with you is based on "science" <u>not</u> diet or marketing hype. I encourage you to research on your own. Research the supps mentioned, especially the 5. Research the clinicals on serotonin and its relation to carb cravings, binge eating, depression, insomnia, ADD, etc. I've also listed several books and websites at the back of this book where you can find further information.

<u>HUMBLING UPDATE:</u> Another move across country, starting my life over yet again, endless challenges of marketing my book, and well, all that stress took its toll. Never would

I believe I'd experience anxiety/panic attacks, but there they were, the worst emotional breakdowns ever. My vitals were soaring. All the while, the most awful thoughts raced through my weary mind. I knew what a lifetime of stress, which can cause high levels of cortisol, can do to the mind/body. I also knew I hadn't been as faithful in taking my hormones (and supps) since I left CA. As helpless as I felt, my saving grace was that I was praying it was due to them being low, particularly my progesterone, as it plays a major role in our emotions. When my blood tests came back, my hormones weren't just low, they were flatlined. I wasted no time getting back on them. I also got back on my supps, upped my 5, and added more magnesium. Though I felt better, the anxiety was still simmering below the surface. So, more research. I focused on how anti-anxiety drugs work. I found that GABA (gamma-aminobutyric acid), is the main inhibitory neurotransmitter in the human cortex, referred to as the "anxiety" amino acid. It works on the same principle as Xanax. Within days of taking 500mg at night, that overwhelming, terrifying sense of panic was gone. Equally important; absolutely avoiding all sugar, high GI carbs, etc. Moral of the story? My suffering, forced me to research much further. As such, I'm helping my clients alleviate their anxiety and panic attacks even more quickly, and still, without drugs.

Feeling anxious? Panicked? You're not alone.

UPDATE: BIOIDENTICAL HORMONE WARNING

Since I've been in the Atlanta area, I've been unable to find a doctor who truly knows how to properly test hormone levels and/or successfully treat the many symptoms of menopause. Because millions of women are now entering menopause, this has become a huge money maker for many doctors. Unfortunately, however, most are not trained in anti-aging medicine. Just because they have a medical degree, they somehow feel they're qualified to offer bioidentical hormones. They are not. In addition, they charge $450-$600 per visit/three times a year. That does not include the actual hormones or testing.

My first hormone doctor in ATL was a man. He was board certified in anti-aging. But, as a man, he couldn't truly empathize with me, as a female. And, he was lost on how to help me with my ongoing anxiety. My own research showed estrogen dominance contributes greatly to anxiety, plus, many other menopausal issues. More disturbing yet, every time I was tested, my hormones were always low. So what was it all for then?

I changed to a female ob/gyn who offered hormone treatment. I warned her ahead of time that I am extremely sensitive to any and all meds, OTC, changes in delivery of hormones, etc. She still insisted, though, on changing my hormones and their delivery. Within days, my BP and HR were soaring. Worst of all, when I knew something was wrong, I called to talk to her, to get help. They said I had to make an appointment. I told them it was urgent. Sorry, make an appointment. After training clients, I actually drove myself to the ER where my BP climbed to 177/99 and HR at 110. (My HR is never higher than 40-45.) When her office finally called me back, I told them I was in the ER. All the nurse could say was, "Oh, sorry to hear that."

The doctor never called me. She never cared enough to check on me. I finally heard from her a month later with a letter. *A letter?* She denied any wrong doing. In fact, she blamed my reaction on my "sexual lubricant." What? She couldn't be serious! My vitals were up for days. The last thing I was interested in was s-e-x. I moved onto yet another doctor, hoping she could help me. She put me on a synthetic hormone versus bioidentical. Again, my vitals soared. This doctor apologized profusely, blamed it on my adrenals, but I was done. No more.

Bioidentical hormones still serve a purpose. Maybe one day I'll try them again for all the benefits they offer menopausal women. In the meantime, I'll do what I can to remain healthy: strong bones, lean body mass, mental capacity, heart, etc., by eating healthy, weight training, plenty of water, sleep, and supps. Since I've stopped taking the hormones, my anxiety is much better by simply avoiding all high GI carbs, taking the 5 faithfully, and enough of the right form of magnesium. GABA, if and when anxiety rolls in.

TO HOPEFULLY INSPIRE: No hormones for the last six months or so. Age 57 here, and, I train just two to three days a week. I still have hope . . .

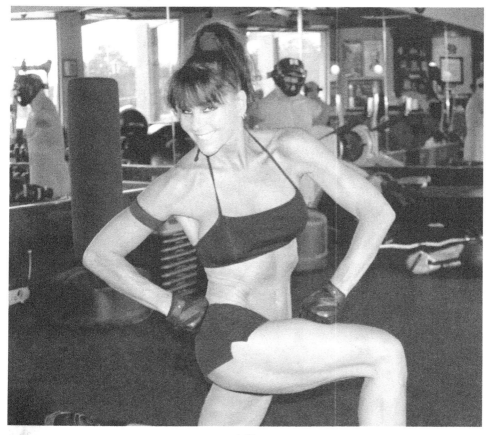

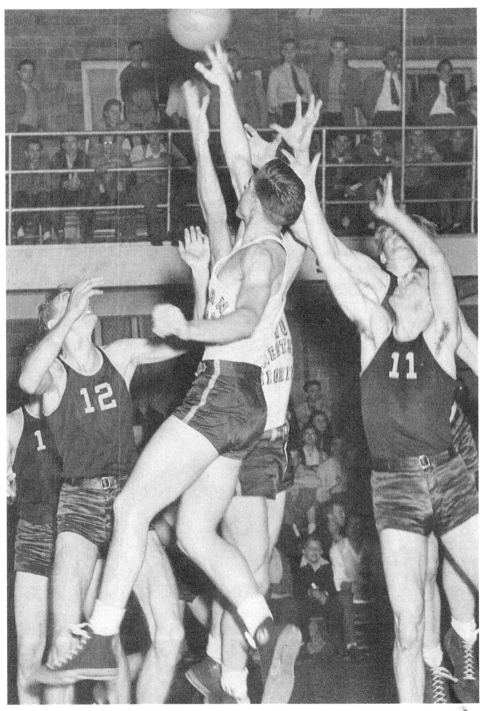

25

GENES...
Use 'em or abuse 'em

You've shared so many amazing things with me, but I must ask, with regard to achieving this extraordinary health you speak of, isn't it really more about some people just having good genes?

No, and please don't allow yourself to fall for this myth. If you feel you were somehow shortchanged in this department, just push yourself harder. Clearly, some people have better genes than others. So what. I feel I am extraordinarily blessed when to comes to my genes, starting with my beloved grandmother. Harriet Vander Molen, born August 1,1897, was an amazingly strong (physically, mentally, emotionally, and spiritually), independent, courageous, and passionate Dutch woman. One of my earliest memories as a young child was waking up in the warm and loving embrace of my grandmother's arms. Rising with the sun, and before she even got out of bed, she'd do a couple of dozen leg lifts. Followed by a variety of arm exercises, then twisting away on "Trim Twist," a flimsy wooden platform to help keep her waist trim. (Or so she hoped.) Twenty minutes later, she'd go downstairs to have a Shaklee protein drink and read her Bible and daily affirmations. Little did I know how advanced she was. Little did I realize that my grandmother was fueling her body, mind, and spirit for the day.

What a great way to live life!

After her breakfast of herbal tea, oatmeal with heavy cream, side of prunes, home-baked bread with real butter, she'd shower and then off to work. She was a personal caregiver and, among many things, she had to physically lift her patients numerous times on any given day. Being a widow for as long as I could remember, my grandmother worked happily into her seventies. After she retired, she traveled the world. She came to visit me several times in Florida, always eager to seek another adventure with me. (At only 22, I had plenty.) At 82, my grandma used to climb up on the roof of my apartment, boosting herself up two very tough ledges just so she could sunbathe topless with me. However, one of my favorite memories was when we were invited out on a 110-foot yacht for a sunset cruise to sip champagne and dine on fresh lobster. No big deal for most. But considering my grandmother didn't know how to swim, she was deathly afraid of the water. So what! She threw caution to the wind just so she could enjoy the moment with me. Oooh, how I miss her loving and adventurous spirit. She truly was amazing. Her motto was simple: *Try anything at least once!* What a great way to live life. She was also a very passionate woman. In her late eighties, she had men 20 years her junior, and some married, seeking her affections. Talk about genes. In fact, up until the day she died, men adored her. We should all be so fortunate to be that desired at that age, or any age, for that matter.

145

My grandmother lived to be 93 years young and had nothing more than a touch of arthritis. She easily maintained her figure and her mental health. At 5'9", she was proud of being able to keep her weight at a slender 125 pounds. Plus, I never knew her to be sick. She never took any pharmaceutical drugs. It was about a "healthy lifestyle." If she were alive now, she would never give into all these drugs. My grandmother knew, even way back then, that eating R-E-A-L food, and never skipping meals, was essential to good health. She took pride in growing her own garden. She rarely, if ever, drank alcohol, enjoying maybe a small glass of red wine on the holidays or at a Sunday dinner. She also knew the tremendous health benefits of a power nap. Her rewards for this lifestyle were living a long, happy, healthy, and fulfilled life. As I reflect, she really did live an amazing life. I'm forever grateful for that loving relationship. (I realize, happily, I have become my grandmother.)

My grandfather Cornelius Gilman, born September 2, 1891, was a strong, determined Dutchman. I never knew him, as he, sadly, died of colon cancer at age 69 when I was just a baby. Nevertheless, he and my grandmother passed their genes on to my father.

My father Frank at 6'2", 185 pounds, with black hair and hazel eyes, was a gorgeous, all-natural, all-American athlete at Western Michigan University. In addition to his handsome good looks, he was a kind, soft-spoken, hard-to-anger, humble man, the type of man women adored. Similar to others of his generation, he smoked cigarettes early on, but eventually quit. He ate exceptionally healthy based on the AMA's recommendations back then, which of course, was low fat. Nevertheless, he never ate junk food. Just like his mother, I can't recall my dad ever being sick. If he was, it never slowed him down. He went to work every day, was never late coming home. He never stopped to hang with the boys, never disrespected his wife or ignored his responsibilities as a father. He'd religiously have two martinis with my stepmother before dinner so as to unwind. To bed by 11:30. Up by 7:15. This pattern never varied. My father was professionally driven, running his own successful lithography business. I'm grateful that he took tremendous pride in making sure his children were well provided for (not pretentiously), while quietly encouraging us to follow our own unique path.

On the weekends, my dad used to love to do yard work, shoot hoops, swim, snowmobile, and water ski. Now, at 81, my concern is where he and my stepmother carry their extra weight, i.e., at their waistline. Unfortunately, they're still eating a low fat diet, which equals too many carbs. Plus, other insulin stimulating factors. Prolonged high insulin levels lead to numerous health risks far beyond weight gain. While my dad's wise enough to avoid most pharmaceutical drugs, he's taking high blood pressure and a statin. Both of these issues are often due to high insulin. Although he's had a bad back for 20 years, his high insulin levels (and the statin that his doctor has him on) worry me the most. Nonetheless, he still enjoys his yard work, grows a small garden of vegetables, travels, and plays a mean game of golf three times a week (18 holes—and now, at age 82, he's shooting a 78), followed by an ice cold beer with his buddies. He's happy and enjoying his life. (Due to nerve damage, my dad conveyed my many concerns about statins to his doctor. Thankfully, he pulled him off it.) **UPDATE**: After reading my book, and being willing to follow some of my nutrition suggestions, I'm proud to say my dad's lost 18 pounds. He looks fantastic!

With respect to my mother's parents, I only knew them for a brief time. But what I can remember was a lot of smoking and drinking. My grandfather died of a heart attack when he was in his sixties, with my grandmother dying in her early seventies.

My mother Barbara Holcombe suffered from what the American Psychiatric Association likes to call "mental illness." Yet never did I hear of her exhibiting any type of behavior that would warrant such a diagnosis, let alone be committed. If she did, it was only <u>after</u> they put her on heavy meds, which lead to such behavior. Nonetheless, she was institutionalized when I was barely two. Though I never knew her as I was growing up, based on photos and family stories, she was an incredibly stunning, petite, creatively inspired, highly spirited, and very passionate woman of Belgian decent. She and my father had four children. Only when I was in my 40s, was I fortunate enough to spend time with her. I discovered for myself what an amazing woman she really is. Her heart is so kind, reaching out to everyone with such compassion. Her emotions run even deeper. As for her diet, the meals she's fed are old fashioned and LOW FAT, i.e., meat, potatoes, veggie, dessert, skim milk, coffee. For 73, she's done pretty well at keeping her little figure, but high insulin levels are never good. My other concern is that she smokes way too many cigarettes, drinks far too many sodas, and occasionally she's even given a cocktail. *And why should this concern me?* Because each, and, most assuredly, the alcohol, play a huge role in further depleting her serotonin, not to mention the potentially deadly interaction of the alcohol with her meds. This is distressing, because she's on these meds to stabilize her depression, yet neither her doctor, psychiatrist, or caregivers are aware of the added risk that each bring.

The saddest part of all of this, however, is how my mother cries to me, saying how sorry she is for not having been there for us—and how hard she's tried her entire life to "be normal." I certainly understand she's on serious narcotics to help balance her mentally/ emotionally, but I cry with her, and for her, because she's more normal than most people I meet on any given day. More upsetting yet, knowing what I know now about purported mental illness/depression, causes thereof, the safe, effective treatments available, etc., I truly believe my mother could have lived a wonderfully fulfilling, happy, and yes, *normal life.* However, her only treatment 50 years ago was mind-numbing, psychiatric, addictive drugs and electroshock therapy. *Talk about destroying one's mind.* Even now, over 10,000 people die each year from this alleged therapy. The drugs have somehow become more acceptable. But be not mistaken. They're still mind-altering, addictive, and deadly. These doctors stole my mother's life. They also robbed me (and my siblings) of our mother.

For those who should doubt just how evil the majority of this profession was, and is, I urge you to tour the museum at CCHR (Citizens Commission on Human Rights). Let history speak for itself. Let today's headline news stories remind you of what's really going on. As for my mother not being there for us, it wasn't her fault. She's not alone, though, with her demons. My greatest torment is that I waited so long to go see her. I also find it sadly ironic that my path in life would focus on this precise area of science.

So, was I blessed with good genes? Yes and no. My mother was simply, and unforgivably, a victim to the fraud set forth by the psychiatric profession, a profession that admits to having financial ties to big pharma. Hmmm...no motive there. Either way, I choose to focus on the positive. Regardless, I could've taken my so-called good genes and abused them. It's the same with you. Our genes aren't a free ticket to good health or an attractive body. What truly matters is what we do with our genes. Once again, if you feel you were shortchanged, *please do not give up*, no matter your goals. Push yourself harder. Beat the supposed odds and make yourself proud.

I agree with you. It's just that I hear many of my friends use this as an excuse.
Yes, there are those who would rather find an excuse than face the challenge, a challenge that is well worth your efforts, a challenge that can be life-changing. Another common excuse is that it's "too late." Good news, people. It's <u>never</u> too late to start working out and living a healthier lifestyle! As a matter of fact, because we lose a quarter of a pound of muscle each year after age 30, which then changes our total body composition, you need now, *more than ever,* to start some sort of exercise program.

Is this why I'm suddenly gaining weight, even though my diet hasn't changed?
Generally speaking, yes. When you lose muscle mass, you naturally increase fat stores. Once this shift happens in your body composition, gaining weight is inevitable, and sometimes at an alarming rate.

Can't I just join a gym and do it on my own?
Of course. You can also opt to train at home. But keep in mind, the only thing worse than not working out, is wasting your time when you do. For those women who fear getting big and bulky, this is a myth. Women do not have enough testosterone for that to occur, nor will they be lifting the kind of extreme weight required to obtain that size. This is a far too common excuse some women use to avoid lifting weights. First of all, we each have different body types, so you'll train accordingly. Next, a healthy diet is critical to your success in the gym. The only way you'll bulk up is by training <u>without</u> also modifying your eating and drinking habits.

What do you focus on when you train?
When I train, my goal is never about how much weight I can lift; it is, though, about proper form, technique, and consistency. That being said, I still like to feel a burn afterwards, so I tend to lift heavy. I want to share the following story, only so women will better understand how lifting heavy does not equal big and bulky:

I had just turned 40. I began seeing a man who also trained. He encouraged me to start doing free squats. I typically squatted using a Smith machine. Nonetheless, as a woman who never backs always from a challenge, I decided to try it. May I say, I fell in love. I started with the bar (45 pounds), needing to perfect my form. As the weeks went by, I worked my way up to 190 pounds. I then began to warm up with 225 pounds. Within nine months, I was able to free-squat 410 pounds for 6 reps. At 5'11" and 136 pounds, I was squatting over three times my body weight. (This was, by no means, a parallel squat.)

You're kidding? 410 pounds? Why did you push it so hard?

I wanted to see how far I could push my body and mind. You see, working out requires a lot of mental focus, as well. And I love the competition in my head. You don't need to have a partner to compete. You can just as easily compete against yourself. The other reason I pushed myself so hard was because my now ex-partner and I had just signed with Thane, one of the major infomercial companies. Although my physique was already lean and strong, I wanted to see if I could push my body even further. Pushing the squats was part of that. Furthermore, *and in all modesty*, this was a huge accomplishment for me.

More important than any amount of weight, I want you, the reader, to know that during this time frame my partner and I were dead broke. We were desperately borrowing from family and friends to keep our infomercial project moving forward, as well as to simply have enough to put food on the table. Then, once we were signed, we further struggled to raise the funding required to produce the infomercial. It got so bad we were actually living off my Texaco credit card. Through it all, though, no matter how bad it was, no matter if there was enough money to eat or not, my priority was always to train. I would scrape together my last few dimes to pay the daily gym fee of $5. I'd only train two days a week, but I made my extremely limited time there work. It was enough to keep my mind and body strong. Those two little visits each week saved me in more ways than I can possibly tell you. Hence, for all those of you who may claim you can't afford to work out, I must respectfully disagree. You have no choice, but to afford it. You have to take care of yourself, if you want to enjoy the other many wonderful aspects of your life, let alone, be around for those you love and care for.

NOTE: That's my father, Frank Gilman, (Center) 1946, featured on page 152. What an athlete he was.

UPDATE: Sadly, both my father and mother passed away in 2011. Somehow my dad's doctor convinced him to go back on that damn statin. It destroyed his kidneys. I won't lie: I am very upset with my father for going back on that drug. Instead of allowing me to help him, as I do with my clients, he chose the easy way; a pill. However, a deadly pill that tragically ended his life far too soon. As for my beloved mother, she died of COPD. I miss them both.

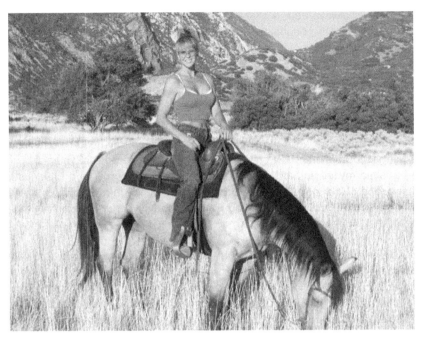

I practice what I preach, decade after decade. Above, 47 years old. Below, 62.

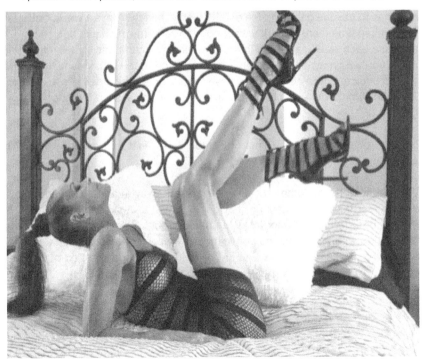

26

EXPECT MORE FROM YOURSELF
Self-care is a must

Expect more from myself? What do you mean?
What I mean is that there are far too many women who, sadly, hide behind their designer outfits, yet never feel comfortable nor confident in a pair of shorts, a sleeveless dress, a bathing suit, and most assuredly, not naked. To those women who think they don't need to workout, because they already wear a size 2, well, I am sorry to disappoint you, but this does not mean you're necessarily healthy. Being healthy means many things; at the very least, it includes a healthy metabolism, heart, and blood chemistry, strong bones, minimal body fat, healthy blood pressure, hydrated skin/body, and having lean muscle mass that is firmly and beautifully sculpted. Now this, is what makes a healthy and attractive physique—for women (and men). Self-care is a must.

Be proud of your body, in and out of clothes.

Ladies, wouldn't you like to be proud of your body, both in and out of clothes? Wouldn't you like to stop camouflaging your problem areas with just the right outfit? Wouldn't you like to be proud of your body and all its little imperfections? *But why stop there?* Wouldn't you like to feel so gloriously sexy that you'd make love with the lights on, or maybe even with the added seduction that comes with making love in front of a mirror? How about eagerly being on top, rather than shamefully hiding under the sheets or your lover's body? Better yet, how about feeling confident enough, ladies, to walk away from your lover, to leave the room <u>without</u> having to walk away backwards? Hmmm? Wouldn't it feel empowering to be proud of your naked body, as you slowly and deliberately saunter across the room? Of course it would.

Okay, forget about all that talk of sex and mirrors. Forget about everyone, but you. My intentions here are pure and simple: I want every woman to be able to stand naked before a mirror and, using an additional mirror, look at themselves from all angles. I want each of you to be able to look at yourself from front to back, side to side, from every possible angle, and truly be happy with what you see. I don't care if you wear a size 4, 8, or 12, perfection is not, I repeat: *Perfection is not your goal.* More importantly, please do not compare yourself to the airbrushed/Photoshop-inspired images you see in magazines. They are not reality. They are a marketing illusion. Instead, I want you to be proud of your naked female body, on <u>your</u> own terms. I want you to be confident in your body, in your appearance, in all that you are. You need to find what truly makes "you" happy. This will inspire and motivate you in many wonderful ways. If you aren't happy with what you see before you, then push yourself harder. *Expect more from yourself.* Refuse to settle for less than what makes *you* happy.

From all angles? Are you serious?
Yes. We are all highly sexual beings. Our brains are our largest sexual organ, but as women, we lose our sexual appetite and insatiable fiery passion when we feel overweight and out of shape. Well, not anymore. Time to change that. Don't let all the silly myths about weight training keep you from trying it. Weight training is about developing long, lean, yet strong muscle and bone mass. That muscle you develop will help burn fat and calories long after you've left the gym. Weight training has also proven to help slow, if not reverse, the signs of aging. *What more could you ask for?* Combine this with a healthy lifestyle and you can once again be that inspiring, sexually stimulating, *self-confident* woman.

But hold on, gentlemen. Not so fast. You are not off the hook here. Far too many of you have also allowed yourselves to get completely out of shape. Statistics verify the alarming pattern of obesity in men, starting as young as 20 and increasing steadily:

Stats regarding obesity in men:
24% age 20-34 • 25% age 35-44
30% age 44-54 • 32% age 55-64 • 33% age 65-74

These numbers are terribly concerning. Though we women certainly have our own issues, with all due respect, gentlemen, do you really think that big belly you're carrying around is attractive to us, let alone healthy? Do you think your 49-inch waist arouses us? What about your once beautifully sculpted chest and strong arms that are now weak and sagging? We women most definitely like a nice firm ass, as much as you men do, so why then did you let yours go soft? It wasn't so long ago, you were eager to get in the gym to make sure you stayed in shape. Suddenly, you no longer care. All those sports you played every weekend have also gone by the wayside. In its place, you find absolute bliss sitting on the couch all day with a beer in hand and a side of chips and salsa. Generally, this change in behavior happens after a man gets married. For some reason, there are men (and women) who fall into a certain comfort level once they're in a committed relationship. He begins to eat and drink more. He works out less. And less. He simply lets himself go. Worst of all, he stops seducing the woman he fell in love with. No longer is he excited to see her at the end of his day. No longer does he give her the affection he once did when courting her. He doesn't understand that making love isn't just in the bedroom. Little does he know there are a million other ways to please the woman in his life.

For those gentlemen who may not be aware, it is not about flowers, candy, or expensive gifts. Though, such gestures are appreciated, it is, rather, about the simplest of things that should be part of any given day. It can be anything from picking up after yourself, putting down the toilet seat, taking out the trash without having to be asked, spending time with the kids away from the house, doing the grocery shopping, helping with the laundry, asking with sincere intent how her day was, and then actually *listening* to her response, be willing to say you're sorry when you're wrong, a passionate hug for no reason (and with no further expectations), a tender kiss on her cheek as you leave the room, a hidden love note, a call in the middle of the day just to say how much she means to you, coming home early and making dinner, drawing her a hot bath with candles lit, to yes, wanting to give her a massage from time to time—minus penetration. While women, without a doubt, want to be sexually desired, we get tired of being sexually pawed at. We want to be acknowledged. Needed. Wanted. Appreciated. Respected. Adored. We want to be thought of. Considered. *We need to feel emotionally connected.* We need to know you love and care about us for far more than what we bring to the proverbial bedroom.

Unfortunately, there are some men who don't realize that to seduce a woman's body, they must first seduce her mind. That, dear gentlemen, is an all-day affair, not just moments before you hope to entice her out of her panties. Consequently, the woman feels unloved, unappreciated, forgotten, worthless, and unattractive. She lashes out. She's hurt. Unhappy. Lonely. Angry. Rarely is the man able to understand her bitter reaction to his inability to express his affections. So, he, too, begins to feel unappreciated and unloved. This fuels an enormous, highly emotional chain reaction between them.

The heavier you get, the less desirable you feel.

This emotional stress that is so often found in relationships severely depletes serotonin. Your brain then endlessly tempts you with the food that will elevate it. The emotional attachment to this food is easy to understand, as the comfort you get from them is often the best part of your entire day. So you keep going back for more. The more you eat, the better you feel. You are also eating to fill the void. You eat to give yourself the happiness, the love you miss. The more you eat and drink to cover what your life is lacking, the heavier you get. The heavier you get, the less desirable you feel. The less desirable you feel, the less sexually inclined you are. Less sexual fulfilment leads to more unhappiness. More unhappiness leads to even more eating. More eating equals more weight gain. No wonder there are so many overweight people, with terribly unhappy and sexless relationships. No wonder both men and women are looking elsewhere to fulfill their emotional needs and satisfy their sexual appetites.

Gentlemen, let me ask you this: Don't you know that women are just as visually stimulated as you are? Don't you think that we want to be with a man who takes pride in his body, naked or otherwise? Don't you know that we want to be with a man who arouses us both in and out of the bedroom? Well, we do. We want to be with a man who loves himself (and us) enough to take the very best care of his body, mind, and soul.

Furthermore, guys, wouldn't you also like to once again look in the mirror and be proud of your naked body? Wouldn't you love to look great in and out of your clothes? Wouldn't it be wonderful to feel strong, confident, and desirable again? Wouldn't you love to feel virile again? Yes, I believe so.

Christine, a friend of mine from CA, admitted that unless she was willing to accept a bit of a belly on a man, she was never going to be able to date again. We laughed about this, but to be quite honest, it shouldn't be so rare to find a man in shape. Nevertheless, no one should have to settle for less than what they truly desire. Now *pleeease* don't go accusing us of being shallow, insensitive women. Women are often painfully reminded that every red-blooded man wants a gorgeous, sexy, and intelligent woman on his arm. Women should want no less. Right? I'm not saying what we want is right for you. Again, no one should have to settle for less than what makes them happy.

Oh, the truth can be tough sometimes! Question is, what can I do for my husband?
Take everything you learn here and put it to use. (Better yet, have him read this book.) Both of you need to make the commitment, once and for all, to take back your health. Stop procrastinating. There is no better time than right now. Healthy levels of serotonin will help you and your husband overcome your carb/sugar cravings, but you will still need to make the effort to live a healthier lifestyle. This includes committing to a regular exercise program and seriously cutting back, if not eliminating, sugar, alcohol, caffeine, cigarettes, and drugs, pharmaceutical and OTC. Eating healthy, getting plenty of sleep, and reducing your stress are all part of this lifestyle, as well. Losing the excess body fat will help you in many wonderful ways. It's also about giving you your sexual life back. To feel passion for the one you love, and then to be able to perform without anxiety, embarrassment, and/or risking your health, can be so rewarding physically, mentally, and emotionally.

How do you feel about the sexual-enhancing drugs targeted toward men?
I believe ED (Erectile Dysfunction) is due to many factors, ranging from poor diet, being 20 pounds above your ideal weight, prescription/nonprescription drugs, especially BP meds, excessive alcohol, smoking, lack of exercise, and so forth. But do you think your doctor would ever consider these factors first before suggesting you take Viagra, Cialis, or any one of the many sexual-enhancing drugs? Of course not. They don't make money that way. To reiterate, the pharmaceutical industry is a business. They are in it to make money. A lot of money, and always at your risk. ED, as with dozens of the other new professed diseases, diseases that are most often created by pharmaceutical drugs themselves, is making the pharmaceutical companies billions of dollars richer. Please keep in mind, though, serotonin controls many things in the human body, libido is only one of them.

Are you saying serotonin controls our sexual desire?
Yes, serotonin controls sexual behavior/desire, but what I'm really trying to convey here is that far too many people allow themselves to get overweight. Among the other many serious health concerns that we've already discussed, one of the first things we lose is our self-respect. Losing our self-respect is *never* good, and once it happens, our sexual passion is not far behind. Eating yourself into oblivion is merely one side effect of this. When it

comes to losing your sex drive, that can become a downward spiral. Reality is: Who wants to get all naked and naughty when they're carrying an extra 40, 50, or 100 pounds? How can you spend a rainy afternoon making love when you're grossly overweight, and thus, barely able to catch your breath? How can you think about sharing a romantic candlelit bubble bath with your lover if you're too heavy to even get into the tub? Who wants to think about making love in front of a mirror if they can't even stand the sight of their own naked body? I know I wouldn't.

Think back to not so long ago, when you were in shape, when you stood tall and proud of all that you were. Remember how confident you were as a single man (or woman) trying to seduce a lover? Think back to when you were proud of your body and how sexy you looked in your clothes—and out of them. Remember how great you felt with a lean, healthy body? Remember when you could wear any outfit you wanted, without having to wear something to cover your butt or stomach? Remember how wonderful you felt and how much energy you had? Remember how physically and mentally strong you felt? Remember how proud you felt as you went about your day?

One of the first things we lose is our self-respect.

Reality is, we each have our own unique health goals. You can achieve those goals, no matter your situation, no matter your age. But are you ready? I mean *really* ready? Are you ready to commit and do what it takes? How badly do you want it? Maybe you think it's too late or that you're too old to change. Maybe you're scared of failing again. Or maybe you simply don't care anymore. Some do not. That's your choice. But if you want to live a long and happy life, one that is free of disease, especially if you want to be around for your loved ones, please make the effort to lose the excess weight. If you're reading this book, I'm going to assume that you sincerely desire a leaner, more attractive, and healthier body and mind. With these comes a healthy sexual appetite.

I'm ready to kick-start my love life! I know my husband would love me to, as well.
To reiterate, sexual energy is so much of who we are as human beings. I'm not saying that life is not complete without it, as I am sure there are many who maybe never liked it to begin with, or who simply no longer want it. But if given the chance to be overweight and out of shape, or to have a body that you're not only proud of, but one that is also sexually arousing, well, which would you choose?

I choose the sexually arousing body!
I hope most would choose to live their life with love, with passion. If that should include sexual intimacy, all the better. For one moment, though, let's stop worrying about the visual aspect of being overweight and making love. I don't want you to think I'm so shallow that all I think about is what someone looks like on the outside. I'm creatively inspired in all aspects of my life, which makes me very visual, not just sexually speaking. That being said, I also need far more than just a gorgeous body. Nevertheless, no matter what your

155

desires are, the human body can be one of the most beautiful things to look at. Please, take pride in yours and see what you can create.

Now I'm definitely ready to start working out, but I need a trainer. How do I know if a trainer is truly qualified?
I'm thrilled you're willing to do what it takes. Just please understand that just because someone is certified does not mean they are qualified. I see way too many trainers who are sloppy, out of shape—some are downright obese. Sorry, but it's true. If I were looking for a trainer, I'd want someone who shows me through their own physique how qualified they are. If they can't do it for themselves, how could they ever help me achieve my fitness goals?

Anything else I can do to make sure I get a good trainer?
Ask around the gym, starting with the manager. Tell them your needs. Don't be shy. You'll be paying good money for a trainer, and you want someone who can produce results, *without* injuries. After they makes their suggestions, I'd spend some time quietly observing those trainers, as they interact with their clients. From there, make an appointment to talk with them to see how they think they can help you. After that, all I can say is you'll need to follow your instincts. Pick the one you feel most comfortable with. Try it for at least 8 sessions and see how you like it. Just remember, if you haven't ever lifted weights before, or if it has been some time since you were last in a gym, take it slowly. Don't let the trainer push you too hard, but at the same time, allow them to do their job. The fact of the matter is, you will be a little sore and you will feel some pain. But trust me, you'll get used to it. Your body will adjust. You'll even begin to look forward to going to the gym. In the meantime, your primary concerns at this point should be that you feel safe, secure, and confident in your trainer's abilities.

With that in mind, I'd like to share the following quick story: A woman once screamed at me with such distaste, "Phoenix, you have the biggest ego I have even seen!" I was stunned by this comment. I was also hurt. First of all, this woman barely knew me. Secondly, I'm rather reserved, not at all boastful. (If I should ever come across as boastful, *please* know it is not my intention, ever. My intentions are only to educate, motivate, and hopefully inspire others.) Nonetheless, I couldn't understand why she'd lash out with such a stinging comment. So, I asked her to please explain why she thought this. She replied, making a reference to the fact I so boldly used my own image on my products and business cards. *Excuse me?* This is what she based such a hurtful comment on? Obviously, I felt the urge to explain that it had nothing to do with my ego, but rather my "body" is my business. It was imperative that I was able to competently reflect my expertise not just through my spoken and/or written word, but also through my *physical* body. I expect others to equally reflect their expertise in their chosen profession. Does this make them egotistical? I should hope not.

Using my image on my products is also good business. Why would I pay a fitness model when I'm capable? As a photographer and one who knows a little something about product branding, it was equally important to start branding myself, at the same time trying to appeal to both sexes through my packaging, which is why the images I choose to use always include both a man and a woman. All of that is trivial; it means nothing compared to my most significant marketing strategy: Inspire others. I want to show the consumer that having a lean, healthy, attractive physique is not exclusive to those who are 20 and 30 years old. My intentions are to hopefully inspire others, no matter their age. So, with a sincere, and, more importantly, humble desire to achieve that goal, I asked Billy, a client and one of my best friends to pose with me. As of my 2nd book edition, he was 57. He undeniably inspired men of all ages. In all modesty, I was 50, hoping to inspire women. And, now, I'm 62 and Billy is 69. We're still lean and healthy.

Your bodies look unbelievable. I'm definitely inspired. You mentioned Billy's a client. I'm curious, was his diet always healthy?
Thank you for the compliments. And, yes, Billy ate remarkably healthy according to what he, and many others, had been told was "healthy" by the FDA and AMA.

Such as?
Billy ate plenty of healthy food, such as chicken, turkey, fish, cheese, eggs, etc., but he also had quite a taste for natural sugars and wannabe healthy fat free carbs. He loved dried fruit, which is nothing more than crystallized fruit sugar. He ate a lot of fat free yogurts, fat free breakfast bars, Fig Newtons, coconut-dipped figs, bananas, grapes, honey, cereal, fruit juice, fat free pretzels, assorted pasta dishes, and smoothies blended with lots of fresh fruit. He also enjoyed a daily Coke at midday to give him that much-needed boost, along with his weekend treat, Milano cookies. As you can see, Billy's carb choices were mostly from natural sugars, but they were high GI carbs. To make matters worse, drinking those carbs in a liquid form (smoothies, fruit juice, etc.), affected his insulin levels much quicker and more dramatically. (I hate to admit it, but while I easily avoided the dried fruit, fruit juice, and yogurts, as they gave me such a crazy sugar buzz, I did enjoy pretzels. *And why not?* After all, they were "fat free." Only now do I realize why I felt so bloated, thirsty, and fat after I ate them.)

Did Billy have weight issues?
No. But, as any man knows, no matter how hard you try, no matter how great the shape you're in, those love-handles can still be a problem. Billy was no different. It wasn't a big problem, but when he was eating all those sugar-laden carbs, they'd go right to his waist. If you want to know how well your diet is working, just look at your waistline. Women generally carry their weight in several areas, from their hips, buttocks, and stomach. Men tend to carry their excess weight in their stomach and chest. Please understand, though, that you may not necessarily reflect this weight gain right away, if ever. But know this; damage is certainly being done to your body and brain.

In all modesty, I'd like to say that since Billy has combined my nutrition program with his dedication both in and out of the gym, he has lost all desire and cravings for those high GI carbs. This, subsequently, helped him gain far more lean muscle mass, while greatly reducing his body fat. He's also significantly improved his blood panels.

Are you saying that 5-HTP helped control his cravings for these carbs?
Yes. Once again, controlling the cravings equals less insulin spiking. Less insulin equals less fat stored, and more fat burned. All of this equals a much leaner, healthier body.

Does Billy have any other bad habits?
I have only two concerns with Billy. First of all, he eats way too many protein bars. While I know he genuinely believes his preferred bar is a healthy choice, because the packaging claims a mere 2 net carbs, they are a perfect example of product deception. In addition to the excessive 240 calories per bar, the manufacturer hides their exorbitant amount of sugars in the glycerine and sugar alcohols, which, by the way, add up to 24g of carbs. A far cry from their professed 2g.

My second concern is Billy's love of caffeine. Maintaining his serotonin levels, combined with my nutrition advice, has helped get him off all those numerous other insulin-producing carbs, which has, subsequently, led to much healthier blood tests, yet Billy is not ready to give up this habit. He, along with a lot of other men, love the buzz that comes from caffeine. Even though I've begged him to at least just *try* decaf, he refuses. Nonetheless, Billy has made so many other extraordinary changes I leave him be. (That is, until tomorrow.)

As I said before, we can't be expected to do everything perfectly. After all, it is about moderation and making the best possible choices. It will require effort. Set small goals. Achieve them one by one. Then move on to the next. Remember, healthy levels of serotonin will help control the actual cravings. What's left is merely the "habit." Question is: *Are you ready to drop those unhealthy habits?* Some habits you may choose to hold on to. However, if you aren't happy with the way you look and feel, your unpredictable, stressed-out, depressed mood swings, or your inability to be intimate—well, then, this is where all those little things add up. Are the protein bars, flavored lattes, cocktails, fried chicken, cookies, crackers, sodas, or french fries really worth it? I hear so many people say they don't want to give up their pasta, chocolate cake, potato chips, wine, etc., but they need to realize that their professed emotional attachments to these carbs are false.

What do you mean it's false?
It's false, because once you elevate your serotonin, your brain will no longer push you toward those carbs. You will no longer desire them. Best of all, you will not miss them. That love affair will no longer serve you well. Now, if on occasion, you still want a treat, go ahead. But the actual *craving* will be long gone. Look, I encourage you to live as healthy a lifestyle as possible. How far you want to take it is entirely up to you. I suggest you at least pick your treats wisely.

UPDATE: After years of gently nagging poor Billy about the health risks associated with stimulants and the fact it's nothing more than a habit, since by boosting his serotonin his actual cravings were gone, Billy has *finally* given in. It's been two full weeks since he's had any coffee. Other than feeling a bit off for the first few days, he says he feels great, with a lot more energy. He also lost a quick few pounds. I told him that without all the water retention due to the insulin constantly being spiked, he would get even leaner than he already is. In addition, he's finally decided to listen to my concerns regarding protein bars. You have no idea how long I've bugged him about both. I am so proud of him.

A lesson to be learned here: Billy's probably the closest one to me and my research, but it shows you just how independent people can be. They have to find their own way, and do it in their own time. But, as long as they make the effort, this is what matters in the end. To reiterate, I don't expect Billy, or anyone else, to make all these changes overnight. As you can see, some habits can take years to break. But it can be done if you truly have the desire. (**UPDATE:** It's now been 8 months since Billy cut out caffeine and protein bars. Not only is he leaner than ever before, but he doesn't miss them one bit. See, habits can be broken, if you're willing.)

And now, Billy kindly insisted on sharing his story, in his own words:
"Over the years, I've struggled, like most, with sugar cravings and finding a balance between diet and exercise. It's not that I was a junk food junky or hopelessly out of shape, I wasn't. I've worked out all of my adult life, but always seemed to carry an extra 5 pounds around my midsection. And for all the working out, and being as active as I am, I wasn't achieving that lean, muscle definition that I knew I could have. I also experienced pretty extreme energy lows in the mid-morning and late afternoon. By 3pm I used to find myself actually having a Coke with a bag of pretzels just to keep my head from hitting the desk. Repeatedly Phoenix would tell me, "You're eating way too much sugar." As a result, I decided to let her help me.

We started by tracking everything I'd consume in a week. I put it into a spreadsheet and broke it down into calories, carbs, protein, fat, and sugar. When we added up the natural sugar (plus the daily soda) that I was ingesting, combined with my carb intake, it was very illuminating. For example, orange juice, bananas, raisins, honey, and yogurt don't sound unhealthy, but they're terribly high in fructose, i.e., fruit sugar. I was eating plenty of them. By eliminating them from my diet and replacing them with low GI carbs and adding more protein, I reduced my sugar intake from an amazing 173g per day to 29g. My carb intake went from 345g per day to 132g. My overall caloric intake went from 3,000 a day to about 2,050, which is right in line for my weight, height, age, and level of activity. My blood panels subsequently became much healthier, too.

With Phoenix's expertise (and the 5), not only was I able to drastically cut back my carb intake without any real effort, but my cravings for all those senseless high GI carbs also just seemed to vanish. No real effort, and I never missed them. This allowed me to get over the obstacles I just couldn't seem to conquer on my own. The end result was an almost immediate loss of about seven pounds around my midsection and a substantial increase in muscle definition. My energy level is now consistent throughout the day, and I have far more energy for my workouts. Furthermore, I was an insomniac for nearly 10 years. I am, however, rediscovering what it feels like to sleep through the night. This is huge for me! I also found my ability to handle stress was greatly improved.

Even beyond those successes, having finally gotten off the caffeine and protein bars, in two weeks, and with no other changes in my diet, I lost another five pounds. Better yet, I finally achieved the results I've worked so hard for.

On Phoenix's 1st and 2nd book covers, I was 53 and 57. At 68, my stats are still excellent; 5'11", 180 pounds, with a 34.5" waist. Body fat is 15%. Blood pressure 120/70. My HDL increased; 41 to 69. VLDL are low at 14. Triglycerides have decreased; 147 to 71. My PSA also excellent. And all, without drugs. I train three days a week. My cardio exists of walking and riding my bike. Everyone needs to learn this truth about living healthy. I can honestly say, I'm feeling better than ever! Thank you, Phoenix, for all you've done for me! You know how much I love you."

UPDATE/COVID: *"Unfortunately, I got COVID in 2020. I was sicker than ever and it lasted for three agonizing months. An endless dry cough and high fever. I truly believe the only reason I didn't die, like so many others, was due to my healthy lifestyle that Phoenix has taught me for nearly 30 years. Over those three long months, I lost 15 pounds and my muscles atrophied. I was weak. My hair was falling out. Though I finally stopped coughing and my fever eventually broke, I was mentally and physically exhausted. I wasn't about to go back to the gym with all the risks of the virus still lingering. Phoenix was gracious enough to train me online twice a week. Within just two months, by combining her nutrition expertise and highly effective style of training, I was feeling much stronger. About seven months later, she gave me back the physique I had prior to COVID—and possibly even better. I finally feel like myself again. I'm back up to 180 pounds, with a 34.5" waist, 15.5% body fat, and I'm now . . . 70 years old. I feel so much better. I can't thank Phoenix enough for helping me get healthy and back into shape!"*

It was my absolute pleasure, Billy. You know exactly how much you mean to me. Thank you for sharing your experience with my readers, both before and after COVID. It was awful to watch you go through that. All the more reason why I'm so thankful you've allowed me to guide you on your nutrition all these years. You are an excellent testimonial, and a perfect example of what one can achieve, if they truly make the commitment. Your story, along with your phenomenal photos, will undoubtedly, inspire men everywhere.

The lesson of the day:
Age is not the determing factor
when it comes to your health and fitness goals.

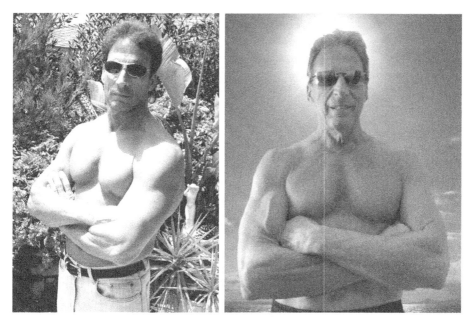

Billy, age 53 & 70. Remarkable!

Phoenix, age 59

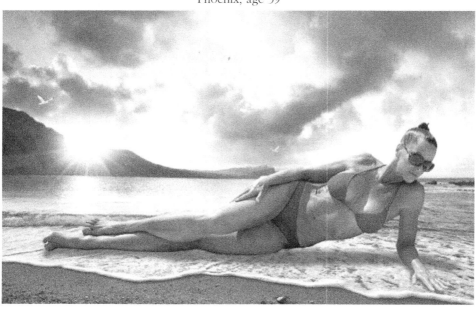

It is imperative that I practice what I preach.
Age 57. Waist: 26 inches

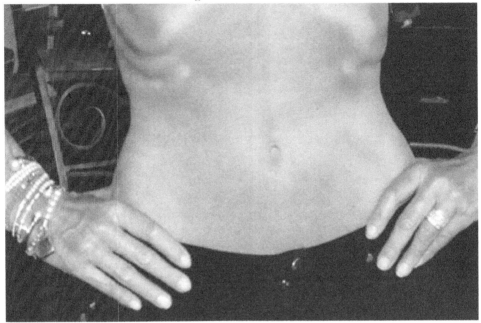

Billy, age 64. Waist: 33 inches

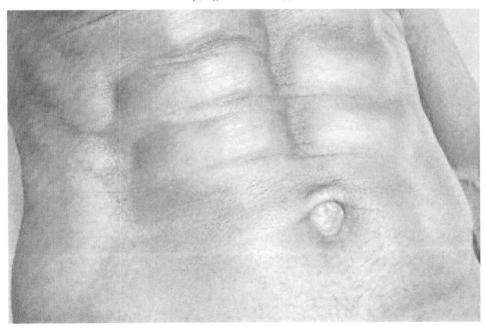

27

"GOT ABS?"
One of the biggest weight loss myths

No matter how much ab work I do, my tummy is still fat! Please explain it to me again.
This is one of the greatest myths perpetuated throughout the diet/fitness industry. I could do a 1,000 crunches with a client and their tummy will not get any leaner or flatter. I will make their core stronger, but not leaner. *Why?* Because your stomach is a direct reflection of your D-I-E-T. If you're still eating carbs that trigger your insulin, then your stomach will not get leaner, nor will you be any healthier.

No wonder my tummy never gets any leaner, or flatter!
The muscles in your abdomen are small strips of muscle. Hence, they do not burn a lot of fuel, i.e., body fat. It's the larger muscle groups; glutes, legs, back, and chest, that burn a lot more fuel, which means your body will, subsequently, be burning a lot more body fat. Plus, you can <u>never</u> out train a poor diet. 80/20 rule: 80% nutrition. 20% training.

Getting a lean, flat stomach is what most people strive for, but, sadly, one of the biggest myths told about getting healthy, and why so many people give up when they do finally join a gym, especially women, because it's also terribly unfamiliar to them. They want to lose the weight, but don't really know how. So, like millions of others, they join the local gym. They go in excited for change, walk on a treadmill for 10 minutes, while reading a book, followed by five minutes of various ab machines, and then walk out thinking they trained. They did not. Their body never changes. They're still eating the same unhealthy carbs that are triggering their insulin. They have no idea how to train. (This often applies to most men, too.) Thus, after a few months, they're extremely frustrated by the lack of results. They quit. They go home and eat some pizza, washing it down with a large soda. They do nothing else, until the next new year rolls around. The cycle repeats again and again.

FACT: Your stomach reflects not only your diet, but also DISEASE within the body. Focus on reducing your waist and insulin gauge. This is when your health will improve in so many extraordinary ways. This is the science behind achieving optimum health.

FACT: You have to have muscle mass to burn body fat. The more lean muscle mass you have, the more body fat you will burn—and the healthier you will become.

FACT: Cardio is a muscle depleting exercise. Stop beating up your body, organs, joints, etc., with all that running. Make your body work for you 24/7 by building lean muscle mass. Muscle is metabolically active. It will burn body fat 24 hours a day.

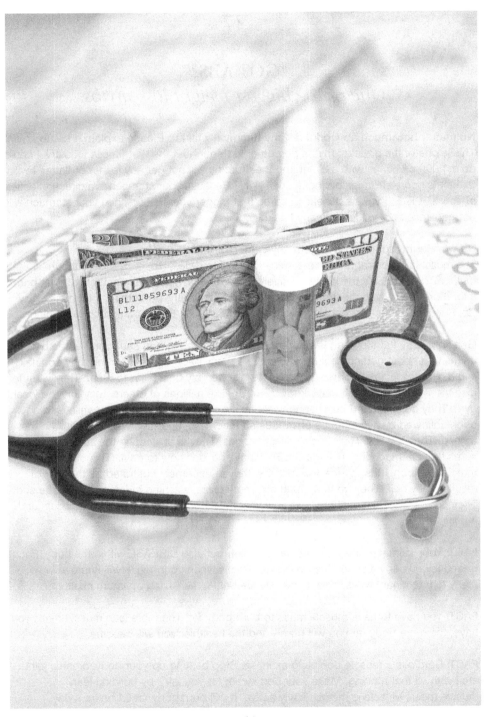

28

PHARMACEUTICAL DRUGS & THEIR SIDE EFFECTS
Weight gain, depression, heart failure, new disease, even death

Drugs, everywhere. How do they promote weight gain?
Pharmaceutical drugs, as well as nonprescription drugs (OTC meds, and that includes ordinary cold meds, pain relievers, etc.) are substances <u>foreign</u> to the body. They're not natural. They're chemicals and poisonous. These drugs will, at bare minimum, trigger insulin. High insulin levels, as you recall, will lead to harmful cholesterol panels, increased water retention, and fat storage. These drugs will also deplete serotonin.

All pharmaceutical drugs deplete serotonin?
Yes, and although serotonin is a major neurotransmitter that controls many vital things within the body, side effects from these drugs can be far more serious.

They encourage weight gain (and depression) due to the fact these drugs deplete my serotonin, hence, causing cravings for the carbs that trigger insulin. Is this correct?
Yes. But remember, these drugs themselves, trigger insulin, causing all sorts of other health problems. Taken long enough, these drugs can actually create new disease and perpetuate the very illnesses they are designed to so-call cure.

Our midsection is an excellent way in which to gauge how healthy our diet is, but it also reflects side effects from various drugs. Hence, one of the first things I ask a potential new client is, "Which pharma drugs are you taking?" After all, this is one of the biggest factors contributing to why people either begin to gain weight, or why they can't lose weight, even though they're working out and eating well. (Observation: Did you notice I didn't bother asking "if" they were on any such drugs? The reason is, because there are very few people who aren't on at least two, three, or even more drugs. Worst of all, their doctors scare them into believing they need to be on a lifelong drug regimen.)

Unfortunately, some refuse to acknowledge the drugs may be a problem. They find it easier to blame me, or another health professional. These people are also the ones who tend to believe their physicians are God. They refuse to question why their bodies are suddenly so bloated, why they're so depressed, blood pressure climbing, and suffering from yet another illness every time they turn around.

I thought these drugs helped cure disease?

Hardly. Appallingly, this is what the drug companies would love for us to believe. They mislead us into believing their drugs will cure us. This is not true. I repeat, *this is not true*. Pharmaceutical drugs are not designed to heal or cure disease. Even if you can begin to afford these outrageously expensive drugs, they're designed for, and only capable of, targeting and <u>masking</u> the symptoms of disease. Supplements and/or herbs, on the other hand, have been used successfully for centuries in healing numerous ailments. Plus, no prescription is needed, little to any side effects, and they're affordable.

Pharmaceutical drugs do <u>NOT</u> cure disease.

Are there other drug concerns?

Too numerous to mention. All one has to do is listen to the disclaimers found at the end of drug commercials. Though they're stated way too fast for complete clarity, the drug companies and the FDA themselves are fully aware their drugs are most often dangerous, if not deadly. (This was recently proven by the Vioxx scandal.) But don't believe me or trust these self-promoting advertisements. Do yourself a favor and buy a PDR and use it faithfully as your guide. Also, go to the FDA's own website and research the various, and most often life-threatening side effects, that come with any given pharmaceutical drug. Review the many lawsuits that are filed against the largest names in the pharmaceutical industry.

A perfect example is Lamisil. It's patented and produced by Novartis. Lamisil is a highly recommended drug to help get rid of simple nail fungus. But—*are you aware of the side effects from this drug?* Besides nausea, changes in vision, blood problems, diarrhea, etc., it can cause liver damage and complete liver failure. This is based on reports from the FDA themselves with regard to lawsuits brought against this drug. Yet these side effects are considered *acceptable* by the FDA. It is marketed freely to the public without any regard for those it will harm. What I find equally disturbing is how Novartis advertises this particular drug. They use funny-looking cartoon characters with even funnier little voices, showing them attacking and crawling up under the nails. They make it seem so harmless, cute, and actually inviting to the consumer. Don't be fooled by this marketing strategy.

Liver damage or complete liver failure just to get rid of some fungus?

Shockingly, these are very typical side effects that are associated with pharmaceutical drugs, both prescription and nonprescription. Another quick example is Nexium, the Purple Pill. This drug, which is touted every other minute via TV advertisements for treating Acid Reflux, has no less than 100 potential side effects. I had to laugh as I read the list of declared rare, but nonetheless, potential side effects. The side effects listed actually utilized almost <u>every</u> <u>single</u> <u>letter</u> of the alphabet, and sometimes repeatedly.

WARNING TO PARENTS: Considering a staggering 10 million children have been diagnosed with ADD/ADHD, *which is merely a side effect of low serotonin*, doctors are only too eager to prescribe drugs to treat them, primarily Strattera and Ritalin. I have to ask:

Are parents unaware that these psychiatric drugs are addictive, mind-altering substances, more potent than cocaine? Are they unaware that these drugs come with serious, life-threatening side effects for both kids and adults? Side effects from Ritalin can produce a calculable set of symptoms, including loss of appetite (even malnutrition), tremors, muscle twitching, fever, convulsions, migraines, irregular heartbeat and respiration (profound/life threatening), anxiety, restlessness, paranoia, hallucinations, and delusions, excessive repetition of movements, and formication (a feeling of bugs or worms crawling under one's skin). More frightening yet is that typical side effects can include addiction, abnormal heartbeat, nausea, decreased appetite, insomnia, sexual side effects, liver and heart failure, to suicidal thoughts and behavior. One child actually attempted suicide during the Strattera trials. The FDA is well aware of these risks, but they are, again, considered "acceptable." *Still not convinced how dangerous these drugs are?* Here are the side effects/warnings off the FDA's own Web site regarding Strattera: Weight loss/slowed growth, impaired motor skills, upset stomach, decreased appetite, nausea, vomiting, dizziness, tiredness, mood swings, constipation, dry mouth, insomnia, sexual side effects, problems urinating, menstrual cramps, liver damage, to suicidal thoughts and actions.

The ADD/ADHD scam set forth by the Psychiatric Association

The FDA finally issued a health advisory on Strattera after evaluating Eli Lilly's clinical trial data, data that showed it was <u>increasing</u> suicidal thoughts and behavior in children (at 4 per 1,000). Considering the millions of kids on this drug, this is huge. Even one is too damn many. But, instead of pulling this deadly drug off the market, the FDA simply demanded that Lilly add a black-box warning. It will state: "This drug increases suicidal thoughts among youths." This is insane, if not intentional homicide. Parents, please stop letting your doctor drug your kids. You need to remember that your child's diet plays a *critical role* in their mental/emotional state of mind, as well their ability to focus. Based on what you've learned here about serotonin and 5-HTP, it's <u>not</u> necessary to risk their lives with these drugs. How pathetically ironic that parents lovingly teach their kids to "Just Say NO to Drugs"—all the while the medical industry is drugging them at an alarming rate.

Furthermore, let's all pause for a moment and quietly reflect: Have we all so quickly forgotten what it was like to be a child? Have we forgotten that, as a child, just by the pure nature of being a child, we all probably suffered from so-called ADD/ADHD to some degree? And, while diet indeed plays a crucial role in how children behave, they have a ton of energy that is not easily harnessed. So, instead of letting your kids watch TV or sit at the computer, they need to be encouraged or, if need be, forced out to play, and I mean P-L-A-Y for hours on end. In addition, do not waste another moment in getting them to eat healthier.

Increases suicidal thoughts and behavior? The side effects are far worse than the questionable condition. Why would anyone take the chance?
Exactly. I am once again astounded by what the FDA considers safe to put into the marketplace. Then you wonder why those of us in the alternative healthcare industry get

outraged when the FDA, FTC, and drug companies feverishly campaign to destroy us, or even shut us down completely. While they attempt to frighten the consumer away from buying dietary supplements, tens of thousands are dying each and every year from their "FDA-approved" drugs. Again, don't take my word on any of this. Buy yourself a PDR and review it. You'll be horrified to discover what the drug companies and FDA consider safe and acceptable. To help protect you and your family, you should use the PDR as your guide for any and all medications considered.

This is outrageous. Why is this allowed?
We should all be asking this *exact* question and equally demanding an answer from the FDA, FTC, AMA, drug companies, and our own doctors. Dare to question the incestuous relationship between these agencies. Dare to write your congressional representative and senator. Dare to hold these government and medical agencies liable.

Believe me, I'll start asking. I've also noticed there are suddenly so many new diseases.
You're right. There's a new purported disease discovered nearly every six months, ranging from ADD (Attention Deficit Disorder), AR (Acid Reflux), to ADHD (Attention Deficit Hyperactivity Disorder), to even Adult ADD (Adult Attention Deficit Disorder), to every type of anxiety/depression disorder. And then there's IRS (Insulin Resistance Syndrome). The headlines scream: *"The Newest Silent Killer!"* Hmm, no scare tactics involved here.

The real answer as to *why* we're suddenly being bombarded with so many new diseases is simple, yet terribly frightening: The pharmaceutical industry, selling over $511 billion worth of drugs each year, is BIG BUSINESS at its worst. They're not about to stop searching for more ways to make even more money. One way to achieve this is by literally creating new diseases. Examples: Since when is having a little trouble focusing (ADD/ADHD) suddenly considered a disease? Better yet, since when is a flaccid penis (Erectile Dysfunction) considered a disease? These are, but a few. The list is endless. Yet these health concerns are not diseases; they are *conditions* that are most often due to an unhealthy lifestyle and, more often than not, actually caused by the prescription and nonprescription drugs you're currently taking. They are conditions that can most often be reversed by first getting off all such drugs and medications with the help of a qualified alternative healthcare practitioner, and by making serious changes in your diet and overall lifestyle. Good health will not be achieved by taking drugs.

Once again, the prescription and nonprescription drugs that your doctor continually forces you to take to treat these conditions, will, in fact, create new conditions and diseases in your body. Furthermore, the more "conditions" the pharmaceutical industry can claim as a "disease," the more power and control they will have over that supposed disease/disorder. They get to develop and market even more drugs to *mask* the symptoms of that "newly designed" disease. Even more disturbing yet, is that, once the pharmaceutical industry makes those claims, once they turn that condition into a DISEASE, no one in the alternative healthcare industry can, in any way, diagnose, treat, cure, or simply try to help prevent that particular condition. *Why?* Big business at work, once again. The answer is simple: Greed. The FDA will do anything and everything to keep the power, control, and profits gained from treating any and all illness in the hands of the drug companies.

Considering the FDA is financially supported in countless ways by the actual drug companies, which is unethical, if not downright criminal, they have much to lose. Hence, the FDA works hand in hand with the pharmaceutical industry to annihilate any persons who attempt to threaten their monopoly and profit margins.

Once again, the pharmaceutical industry is NOT designed to cure or heal people. It is a proven fact their drugs are merely meant to target and mask symptoms. The drug companies themselves admit to this. They have, though, brainwashed patients, even doctors, into believing that their drugs are the only effective treatment. Reality is: The pharmaceutical industry is an investment industry motivated *entirely* by the PROFITS of its shareholders. It is about the billions of dollars that are made by patenting their assorted drugs. It is not about curing disease.

What's even more disturbing is that, to expand their market, pharmaceutical companies continually search for new uses for their assortment of drugs. This is a new medical category called "pre-disease." They are scaring otherwise healthy people into believing they need to be on any number of their drugs to help avoid *potential* disease. A few examples of pre-disease drugs that are being heavily marketed are Fosamax and Actonel to prevent osteoporosis. Plavix, a drug promoted to prevent stroke. Or so they'd love for us to believe. But *why* do they leave out the many serious side effects from taking these drugs? I'll tell you why. Because this, along with all their many drug claims, is nothing more than an insidious, self-serving marketing illusion.

Another example: Although aspirin is an OTC/nonprescription drug, Bayer has become the poster child for helping stop heart attacks. Over 50 million people have been convinced that simply by taking Bayer daily, they will either avoid a heart attack, or greatly reduce their risks for having one. *Really?* Where are the unbiased clinical studies to support this claim? Why do they conveniently forget to mention the side effects associated with taking an aspirin every day, i.e., stomach bleeding, kidney damage, even death? It also increases the odds of another often fatal condition; hemorrhagic stroke. Aspirin may offer some health benefits, but why aren't doctors promoting *living a healthy lifestyle* versus having to take aspirin to counter unhealthy lifestyle habits?

The aforementioned drugs are merely the tip of the proverbial iceberg. All one has to do is stay home and watch TV for a day to see that nearly every single commercial is a drug ad. These deadly drugs are cleverly promoted through million-dollar ad campaigns specifically designed to frighten you into going to see your doctor, who will then most definitely convince you that you must be on any number of their drugs. Considering that the majority of people blindly trust the medical industry, these endless fear-based ads are ferociously successful. As far as I'm concerned, based on what I know, and based on many other experts within the alternative healthcare industry, those involved in the drug industry are nothing more than legally acceptable drug dealers. All of them are in bed with the FTC and the FDA. While one hand despicably washes the other, profits for these organizations grow exponentially—and all at our expense.

Worst of all, most people will fall for their deception. Sadly, the elderly are the easiest victims when it comes to these drug peddlers. They, unfortunately, never question their doctor. They so willingly put their very lives in their doctors' hands, only to be abused in the worst possible way. (Two of my dearest friends died due to a plethora of deadly meds.) Don't kid yourself, the AMA is fully aware of how easy it is to manipulate the millions of seniors under their trusting care. That market alone is making them billions. Now, can you imagine the profits to be made off the baby boomers, as we creep into our later years?

Furthermore, one cannot possibly ignore the outrageous costs related to these drugs. The elderly are literally forced to go without food in order to take the drugs that their doctor insists they must take. Millions of seniors are going hungry, without heat or air condition-ing, in an attempt to buy these drugs, drugs that, instead of healing them, are, in fact, killing them quicker. I have to ask: *Where will this end? How can this be allowed? Does no one care? Are we all so damn busy, so completely unaffected that we just turn our heads away and pray we never get sick?*

Life Extension magazine recently wrote a powerful article speaking out against the whole FDA/drug company scandal. They included a chart outlining the most popular drugs and their costs, compared to supplements, markups, etc. Example: Xanax, is a tranquilizer used for treating and relieving anxiety, with a dosage of a mere 1mg. The cost of the gener-ic active ingredient for 100 pills is only $0.02, while the drug companies sell it for $136.79. The drug companies legally allowed markup for this drug is a staggering 569,858%.

As previously mentioned, another successful strategy to broaden the reach of Big Pharma is to create new diseases with their drugs. Because these drugs only mask symptoms, most, if not all, of the drugs that millions of people are currently taking for one health problem or another, will be the cause of many new diseases. This is a direct result from the drug's long-term side effects. Perfect example: One very common side effect from taking any pharmaceutical drug is the loss of sexual desire and/or function. Rather than address the underlying reasons why their patients have suddenly lost all sexual desire or ability, it's far more beneficial financially to the drug companies to simply create a N-E-W disease. This particular new disease is, again, ED (Erectile Dysfunction). Another example: Cholesterol-lowering drugs. Numerous studies show that these drugs are known to actu-ally increase the risk of developing cancer. The list is endless and atrocious.

With regard to how many drugs some people are taking, as well as how drugs can create new disease, I felt it was important to share this news story: The makers of Botox, pharmaceutical company Allergan and Dr. Arnold Klein, a Beverly Hills dermatologist, were sued by Mike and Irena Medavoy. Their suit claims Irena was treated with Botox to help ease her migraines, but instead became extremely ill, suffering from continued migraines, fever, respiratory problems, and hives. Some symptoms eventually subsided, but many allegedly did not. While this is a story well worth following on its own, my focus was drawn to the evidence brought forth by the defense team. They claimed that the dozen-plus pharmaceutical drugs Irena was taking, in addition to her Botox treatment, were the underlying cause of her symptoms, not the Botox. I was stunned when the lawyer read the number of drugs she was on. Literally, no less than a dozen, and they ranged from antidepressants, several for migraines, anxiety, insomnia, etc. More alarming was that the Medavoys were not even remotely aware of the side effects that were common to these assorted drugs.

Knowing what I know about the effects of taking just one pharma drug, I can't begin to imagine how the excessive amount of drugs are affecting her body and mind. At bare minimum, one of these drugs alone will deplete her serotonin, yet she's taking nearly a dozen. No wonder she's depressed, suffering from migraines, body aches and pain, unable to sleep, and highly stressed. Reality is, every single drug Mrs. Medavoy is taking comes with harmful side effects, creating a new condition or disease. When she complains of these new health problems, her doctor will simply prescribe another drug, which will create a whole new set of side effects, creating yet another new condition or disease, for which her doctor will, once again, prescribe yet another drug that will cause even more side effects. This is a frightening cycle, a cycle that is perpetual and terribly disturbing.

This is also a perfect example of people blindly trusting their doctor. *Why is it no one questions this?* How can two highly intelligent, educated people such as the Medavoys allow themselves to be so senselessly drugged without questioning it or being in the least bit concerned about the side effects of all these drugs?

I admit it's terribly frightening, but we've been brainwashed to believe that our doctor knows best. Apparently, this blind faith is not in our best interest.
Blind faith is never good. All I ask is that you learn to question your doctor's proposed treatment and do some research on your own. To reiterate, the pharmaceutical industry is a BUSINESS. Their business is disease. It is one of the biggest scams on mankind. The endless promises of health touted by these pharmaceutical companies is not reality. Instead of renewed health, cures, or healing, most often their trusting patients are met with life-threatening side effects, new diseases, even death.

It's one thing if these drugs worked, even with such horrendous side effects, but they do not. To make this matter even more unsettling is the fact that the FDA, AMA, drug companies, and FTC will stop at nothing when it comes to trying to scare people away from alternative, all-natural methods of treatments. You see, the actual survival of the pharmaceutical industry depends on the elimination of any and all alternative health therapies, including dietary supplements.

Please understand, I'm not saying doctors don't have a value. They do. My hope is that you learn to think for yourself. Do NOT take what these doctors say as gospel. Stop letting them put you, and yours, on all these senseless, ineffective, and harmful drugs. Research your options, starting with making sure you choose your physician with the greatest of care. You also need to realize that doctors have a stake in the drugs that are sold to you, their patient. Doctors get huge kickbacks from drug companies, ranging from lavish trips and dinners, free tickets to elite sporting events, golf vacations, etc. Big pharma spends, on average, $15K per year, per doctor, to seduce them into pushing their drugs. *And yet no one sees a problem with this?* Talk about a secure drug deal. (**NEWS UPDATE**: Pfizer paying record $2.3 BILLION settlement for illegal drug promotions.) This is exactly why you must be willing to respectfully QUESTION AUTHORITY. (Same for your vet, dentist, mechanic, lawyer, priest, accountant, etc.)

My doctor is always rushed, barely allowing me to speak. How do I approach him?
Politely demand that your doctor give you a moment to express your thoughts and concerns. Considering they're generally no less than 30 minutes late for our appointments, the least they can do is give us their undivided attention for a few moments, once they enter the room. Do not let their rudeness keep you from getting your much-needed answers. In addition, don't be afraid to question their diagnosis, treatment, medications, potential side effects, etc. After you leave the appointment, go home and research so that you're better informed. Then either make an appointment with a new physician or call your doctor back. Tell him your concerns. Share your opinion. Be considerate, but demand answers. Dare to protect yourself and your family. If you're not satisfied with his response, then insist on getting a second, third, even fourth medical opinion.

Companies that kill for profit? Which corporations do you think of first? Halliburton, Blackwater, Lockheed Martin? Yes, they're on the top of the list, but I'm talking about Merck, Pfizer, Lilly, Philip Morris, etc. Some alarming medical statistics to ponder:

❱ 9,000 people die each year from aspirin, ibuprofen, and naproxen.

❱ 90,000 people die each year due to hospital errors.

❱ 106,000 people die each year from prescription drug side effects. Over the last decade, nearly 8 million have died from these drugs, with 191 million being injured.

❱ 250,000 people die each year when surgery goes wrong.

❱ 300,000 people die yearly from alcohol. 450,000 people die yearly from cigarettes.

❱ Acetaminophen (Tylenol, Panadol, etc.) can cause liver damage. More than 56,000 people visit the emergency room. Approximately 450 die. **NEWS UPDATE**: FDA report urges tougher acetaminophen warning; the risk of liver damage and overdose.

❱ Celebrex has been linked to 10 deaths and 11 cases of gastrointestinal bleeding.

▶ Vioxx, after 5 years and with over $10 billion in sales, has been pulled from the market due to an increased risk of heart attack and stroke.

▶ Rezulin was pulled off the market after 90 cases of liver failure were reported. 63 of these cases resulted in death, 10 required liver transplants.

▶ Bayer Pharmaceutical has voluntarily recalled its cholesterol-lowering drug Baycol, because it has been linked to nearly 40 deaths.

▶ Paxil, an antidepressant drug earning more than $3.1 billion, is addictive, causing severe withdrawal symptoms in consumers attempting to stop taking it.

▶ Eli Lilly has been charged with 300 lawsuits based on the side effects caused by Prozac. Charges allege Prozac can precipitate suicide in patients who are unable to breakdown Prozac's main ingredient, fluoxetine. For over 15 years Lilly has also covered up their own internal findings that those on Prozac are *12 times more likely to commit suicide* than those on another antidepressant! In 1990, Lilly corporate executives convinced their scientists to alter records on doctors' experiences with Prozac. They changed any mention of suicidal thoughts to "depression" and suicide attempts to "overdose." **UPDATE:** In 2007, Eli Lilly won the FDA's approval to put Prozac into chewable, beef-flavored pills to treat separation anxiety in dogs. *Where will it end?!*

▶ Vioxx: The FDA and Merck are under extreme fire as evidence clearly indicates the FDA approved, promoted, and refused to recall Vioxx, even after they knew it was responsible for an untold number of fatalities. Thus far, 160,000 cases of heart attack and stroke have been reported! This is only the tip of the iceberg when it comes to the FDA working hand in hand with the drug companies only for profit! Just as with the Prozac scandal, those involved in this cover-up should be charged with intentional homicide.

▶ Vioxx continued: The FDA has recommended that Merck resume sales of this proven deadly drug. Considering the evidence (the FDA and Merck were both unequivocally aware of the possibility that Vioxx would kill tens of thousands of people, not to mention cause thousands of heart attacks and strokes), how is it possible then, that the FDA would allow it back on the market? *How can this be?* I'll tell you how. It is solely because of corporate greed, because of the billions of dollars Merck (and the FDA) will make from selling this drug. The FDA's statement to support this deadly move claims they believe the number of people who can "benefit" from this drug far outweighs the possibility that others may suffer heart attacks, strokes, or even die. To further convince the public that this move is justified, the FDA is demanding Merck place a black box warning on the package. They're also asking physicians to properly warn their patients of the risks associated with this drug. Oh, please! They can't be serious. Most doctors don't even educate themselves to the deadly side effects of this, or any other drug, and yet they are suddenly going to care enough to warn their patients? I can't believe this rationalization. We've already seen just how many people have died from taking this drug. But the FDA willingly allows it to be sold? This can't possibly be considered acceptable medical treatment.

▶ Celebrex update: Pfizer announced that it has suspended use of its popular Celebrex medicine in a long-term cancer study, because patients who used it over an extended time showed an increased cardiovascular risk. However, the company said that it has no plans to pull the arthritis pain drug from the market.

▶ Naproxen update: Naproxen, sold over the counter by Bayer as Aleve, or in the prescription forms Naprosyn and Anaprox, have been found to increase risks of heart attacks and stroke by 50%! The FDA, though, as with so many other dangerous drugs, refuses to pull it from the market. Instead, they simply recommend the consumer should "consult their physicians and follow instructions on the labels."

This is unbelievable!

Yes, it's hard to believe, but the AMA, FDA, FTC, and drug companies see the previous statistics as nothing more than the "cost of doing business." They also have tremendous influence when it comes to keeping these alarming facts out of the headlines. It was once reported on CNN, and stated by one of the FDA's very own, long-time employees that, "The safety of the consumer is the FDA's lowest priority."

The list is incalculable of horrendous, but apparently acceptable, side effects of prescription and nonprescription drugs, and the other huge money-makers such as tobacco and alcohol. The FDA and FTC conveniently turn a blind eye, never ever considering a ban on these products. *Why?* Because far too many people would lose far too much money. Just the expenditures of the people who get sick from these products and/or drugs are far too big a business to throw away. Instead, these health risks are simply called acceptable and referred to as "The risks associated with treating diseases, with hopes to find cures." *Cures?* They know damn well these drugs will not cure disease. When was the last time we heard of a cure? Polio, maybe. Nonetheless, it's all exceedingly disturbing, as the heartless, profit-motivated drug companies and the FDA clearly have no regard for human life. It is instead all about business and making billions of dollars from human suffering.

WARNING: JAMA (*Journal of the American Medical Association*) reported that the potential dangers of newly FDA-approved drugs are *far higher* than initially believed prior to their going to market. An incredible 20% of new drugs will be labeled "dangerous" or will be pulled from the market. The report went on to say JAMA clearly admits that the safety of prescription drugs is inevitably "tested" on the public. The study concluded with this warning: "Serious Adverse Drug Reactions (ADR) commonly emerge after the FDA's approval.

Tested? *This is insane!* What are we, lab rats?

Yes, we are just that. My suggestion, as well as that of several other health experts, is that if you can't avoid drugs altogether, at the very least, avoid using any new drug. That includes drugs that have been on the market for fewer than five to seven years.

How do dietary supplements rate?

Dietary supplements/herbs have had, on average, fewer than five confirmed deaths per year over the past 40+ years in the U.S. Most of these were due to a single batch of genetically engineered tryptophan produced in the late 1980s. Some were due to ephedra.

I'm both infuriated and empowered by this information. I guess we're all simply too busy with our lives to take notice, that is unless it happens to us. What do you do when you get sick?

Do whatever it takes to stay healthy. Besides a few broken bones, I rarely get sick. On the rare occasion when I do, it's either a cold or flu, both of which I let run their course. I've taken antibiotics, but only as a last resort. (The over-prescribing of antibiotics is another serious issue.) I avoid all other meds, aspirin, cold or pain meds, OTC, pharmaceutical drugs, or otherwise. *Why?* Besides the fact that these medications most often make me feel worse, I also realize that every drug (this includes OTC) I put in my body comes with harmful side effects, some deadly. At the very least, all such meds will deplete my serotonin. This is enough for me not to take them. Nonetheless, I make sure to be fully aware of any and all risks when taking these drugs. So should you. Research the many successful alternative options before you consider drugs or surgery.

Here's another example of how our healthcare system works: When I was finally able to afford health insurance, I was turned down because the carrier I had chosen, Blue Cross, considered me "high risk." *What?* Me, high risk? All because I once had an abnormal pap smear. Even though this is pretty common for women, and even though I took an additional test and paid additional money to resolve this concern, they still refused me coverage. Instead of simply charging me a higher rate, I was flat out declined. My God, if I, with all that I do to stay healthy, in both body and mind, with no health issues whatsoever, cannot get insured, how the hell do most Americans, who are most often borderline diabetic, overweight, pill-poppin', smokin', drinkin', depressed individuals, ever expect to get health coverage? And, if you are fortunate enough to get coverage, the minute you make a claim, the carrier either cancels your policy, or jacks your premiums up so high you can no longer afford it. Either way, they win. It is frightening to realize that health insurance is becoming a luxury that only the wealthy can afford. (I highly recommend you watch SICKO, an excellent documentary by Michael Moore.)

I have no faith in the health insurance system. It is just another shameful scam on the American public. It cannot be counted on. All the more reason why you most definitely need to do whatever it takes to stay healthy. Making sure I maintain my serotonin gives me the ability to do this, by making sure I eat a healthy diet. It keeps me away from sugar, alcohol, caffeine, etc. This is exactly why I encourage others to live a healthy lifestyle starting now, so as to hopefully avoid these medical risks.

Furthermore, with all the purported miracle drugs, why is everyone sicker than ever before? Hmm? *Where are all the healthy people?* By now, you know the answer to that.

Nevertheless, I'd also like to know why the medical industry doesn't promote "Preventative/ Wellness" methods of healthcare instead of simply shoving their deadly drugs down on our throats? Why aren't those individuals who are not burdening the already floundering healthcare system, but instead going to great lengths to prevent illness, compensated in some fashion? People should be able to write off any item and/or service that promotes wellness of body and mind, be it gym membership, trainer, nutritionist, exercise classes, supplements, etc. To those who aren't so easily motivated to get healthy on their own, maybe a tax break might kick them into high gear. Either or, it's a win-win situation, one that actually rewards wellness.

To reiterate, the healthcare system as it's designed today, is all about profits, not about curing diseases. However, as of the Vioxx scandal (with a staggering 100,000 needless deaths) and the many other drugs that are now subsequently being scrutinized, I sincerely hope that this will be the desperately overdue wake-up call that will bring down the FDA and the pharmaceutical industry, as we know them. They need to be held accountable for all the lives they have destroyed, for the trust they have so easily and frighteningly abused, for the endless lies, deceit, and fraud they have perpetrated on the trusting consumer. As I see it, criminal prosecution is a must for all involved. I only wish there were more people like Dr. David Graham, the senior FDA scientist who had the conscience, and the courage, to blow the whistle on his own employer about Vioxx, a drug he knew would kill tens of thousands. Even after he was harassed, intimidated, and threatened by his supervisors, Dr. Graham never backed down and did what was right. Well done, Sir.

Because of all these concerns, and many more, you simply cannot sit in silence. You must be willing to educate yourself, to protect yourself and your loved ones. You must be ready to fight for what you believe, even if that means taking risks. As you know, change doesn't happen overnight. But we can sure as hell get a lot more accomplished when we present our grievances in numbers. Thus, please, take the time to educate yourself. Stop turning a deaf ear and praying it won't affect you. Dare to take a stand on this matter. It could very well save your life, or the life of someone you love.

I rarely meet one who feels as strongly as I do about the outrageous and illegal behavior of the FDA, drug and food companies. (As well as our federal government.) Bill Maher, HBO's host of *Real Time*, is my hero. I applaud him. I respect him for so boldly bringing awareness of these serious issues to his audience. He's a highly informed, passionate individual who has the guts to speak the ugly truths about these terrifyingly calculating agencies. Fellow consumer activist Kevin Trudeau is equally someone who dares to speak up on behalf of the consumer and our constitutional rights; freedom of speech being his primary fight. Trust me, it's a fight well worth taking. Kevin took his grievances one step further. He filed two separate lawsuits against the United States government and the FTC, charging them with "Breach of contract and publishing false and misleading information." His book, *Natural Cures "They" Don't Want You to Know About,* will open your eyes even further to the level of fraud within our government. Though I personally did not find any so-called cures, what concerns me most is his latest diet book that claims you can "Lose 30 pounds in 30 days, and all while eating virtually whatever you want!" Well, you know how I feel about that kind of claim.

Hospital nightmare: 1:30am, Billy called me, needing to be rushed to the emergency room. After waiting 3 stressful hours to simply get him admitted, it then took asking the nurses a dozen times to follow through on his pain meds. Even more alarming, as the nurse was in the midst of injecting him with morphine, she suddenly stopped and asked, "Oh, by the way, you are indeed, Mr. Ciampo, aren't you?" *Excuse me?* She couldn't possibly be serious? Talk about incompetency. She was halfway through giving Billy this drug before she bothered to make sure she even had the right patient. What if this drug had been something other than a pain med? Hmmm? *What then?*

PERSONAL UPDATE: My father started having some health issues. He may need double bypass surgery. During the preliminary tests, a nurse asked him about his lifestyle habits. When he mentioned he enjoys a vodka or two nightly, instead of the nurse saying he should definitely stop drinking during this critical time, she eagerly offered her "favorite summer cocktail" ideas. More incompetence.

Both stories shared are very disturbing. What do you suggest?
My suggestion here is to make damn sure you do everything possible to stay healthy and out of the hospital. If, by some misfortune, you do get sick and have to go, have someone with you watching your back. It could mean life or death. The fact is, 90,000 people die every year due to hospital errors.

Doctor claims: "McDonald's is a healthy choice!"

Another interesting observation: Nearly every nurse, doctor, and medical employee I saw was, at the very least, 30 pounds overweight. As I sat in the cafeteria, I found it further fascinating, and again all-telling, to see the type of carbs not only the staff was eating, but also the visitors. It was another perfect example of watching what happens when serotonin is depleted. With stress being one of the major causes of depletion of serotonin, it's easy to understand why these people were consuming, and with great voracity, nothing but fries, pasta, sodas, bread, donuts, coffee, etc. Their brains were in a frenzy, forcing them to consume whatever food/beverages it would take to elevate this calming brain chemical. And because the staff lives under this kind of stress daily, you can understand why so many of them continually eat this type of food and, consequently, gain weight. I'd venture to guess they probably also suffer from, to some degree, in addition to the cravings, depression, insomnia, anxiety, and/or adult ADD—all symptoms of low serotonin.

Speaking of hospital food, if you believe the medical industry has your best interests at heart, then explain how McDonald's was ever allowed to set up shop in hospitals across the country? *How is that possible?* A doctor interviewed eagerly defended this by saying it was "good for their patients, as McDonald's is a well-known comfort food. It seems to help in the recovery process." I couldn't believe he actually said this, moreover, he expected the public to believe it.

Personal health scare -

Misdiagnosis/Failure to Diagnose/Failure to Provide Adequate Care:
When my creatinine levels became slightly elevated, along with a few cysts on my kidneys, I went to a highly respected nephrologist. Within moments, Dr. N diagnosed me with PKD (polycystic kidney disease), an inherited disease. Even though I had no family history of this "hereditary" disease, he insisted that was what I had. *How could this be?*

At our very next appointment, Dr. N went into great detail about how I just "didn't fit" the typical PKD patient in any regard. Plus, my blood and urine were both benign. Though he couldn't figure me out, he still insisted I had PKD. I was stunned by his statement of confusion, more so, his unwillingness to research further, all the while I was desperate for answers. I thought about going to Emory, to get a second opinion, but to be honest, all the medical professionals and doctors I knew said Dr. N was *the* best.

Though I stayed with him, I began to research endlessly. I even contacted a PKD researcher in CA. He, too, said nothing about me, or my kidneys, said I had PKD. Reality was, there was no family history, my BP was fantastic, no swelling, kidneys were not enlarged and they were working perfectly: I had none of the typical PKD symptoms. However, two years prior, I did drink some extremely toxic water that landed me in the ER. And, as a personal trainer, and one with lean muscle mass, my creatinine levels would also run a bit higher.

For four stressful years, I dealt with this doctor's questionable diagnosis. Yet I continually pleaded with him to find out what was going on with my kidneys. He refused. Do another ultrasound? He refused. He told me not to worry, because kidney function is based entirely on creatinine and mine wasn't that high. I warned him, though, that if something went wrong, he wouldn't know how to help me. And that is exactly what happened.

Years into seeing him every six months, my creatinine suddenly jumped higher. He was alarmed. So was I. And, as I feared, he had no answers, as to why. I was angry. Fed up. He called me to discuss next options. He said he had been doing some research (*really??*), and he thought I might have, "Spontaneous PKD." *What the hell?* He couldn't be serious!

I told him, without a doubt, that I believed my cysts were caused by the poisonous water I drank—and that I did not have PKD, based on the many other factors we had long discussed and agreed upon. Without hesitation he said, *"I agree, Ms. Gilman, you are probably 100% correct. You probably don't have PKD."* I was horrified by how casual he was in admitting he was wrong in his diagnosis. Never had I thought about dying, as much as I had since he labeled me with that disease. His next option? Biopsy. This came with risks. We held off, however, due to COVID.

Months later, as we waited for COVID risks to calm down, I had the most excruciating pain in my left flank. My husband rushed me to the ER. I had a kidney stone. A very large kidney stone: 10x4mm. For over a week, I passed a mere sliver of this huge stone. It felt like a hot drill going through my hip bone! Two surgeries later, two stents, pain meds, extreme anxiety, the worst pain I had ever known, loss of income, and $8,400 out of pocket, I was finally free of the kidney stone and its unrelenting pain.

In summary, I did not have PKD. My multiple cysts (not hundreds, as do those with PKD), were caused by the toxic water I drank. My creatinine was elevated due the kidney stone. *But how did I grow a kidney stone?* Even more negligence. This kidney doctor reviewed my various supps since the first day I saw him. The only one he asked me to stop taking was my kidney cleanse. Yet he never once mentioned the 1,000mg SR vitamin C that I was taking. FACT: *"High doses of vitamin C can increase your risk of the most common type of kidney stone; calcium oxalate."* And, calcium oxalate is precisely the stone I had.

Needless to say, I am absolutely fed up with the medical profession. The level of anxiety this doctor caused me, the pain, the money spent, etc., and for four long years, goes beyond words. He failed me on every front. When I wrote him a letter telling him as much, his reply was: *silence.* I, in turn, filed a complaint against him with the GA Medical Board.

Unfortunately, this is not my only such experience with medical doctors. Not even close. I also hear these kind of stories almost weekly from others. Even more alarming; because a patient has no recourse against such incompetence, this kind of medical malpractice will continue—and without any accountability. Hence, why I do my best to live a healthy lifestyle so I can stay out of the system. I advise you to, please, do the same.

I feel the need to summarize this chapter by restating the following facts:

• The drug companies are *publicly traded* corporations. Their motive is, first and foremost, to make a profit. • The FDA and FTC both work hand in hand with the drug companies. Their priority is not the welfare of the consumer, but rather it's about their profits. • "FDA Approved" means nothing, as drug companies, without hesitation, dangerously manipulate, and thus, falsify their clinical studies to suit their selfish needs. • Prescription and nonprescription drugs are designed to be capable only of targeting and masking symptoms. These drugs do not cure illness or disease. • Taken long enough, prescription and nonprescription drugs will create new illness in the body. They'll also deplete serotonin, leading to depression, anxiety, cravings, obesity, insomnia, ADD/ADHD, ED, heart disease, etc. • If you want to get well and/or remain healthy, try your best to limit all such drugs.

ATTENTION: *If you suffer from an illness or have symptoms of an illness, consult your physician. If you're currently taking prescription drugs or OTC meds, don't stop taking them or replace them based on any information or recommendations appearing in this book without first consulting your medical doctor.*

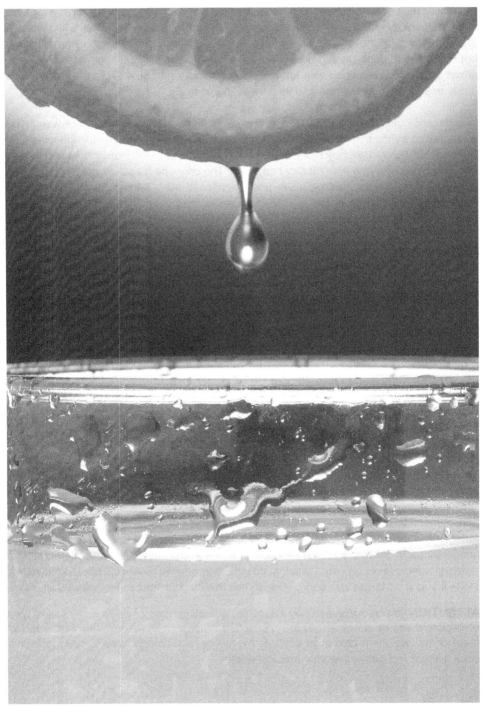

PART II

CARBOHYDRATES
&
THE GLYCEMIC INDEX

All carbohydrates are recognized as sugar by the body.
However, they are ranked quite differently,
based on how quickly they affect blood sugar levels.
This ranking of carbohydrates is called the
Glycemic Index.

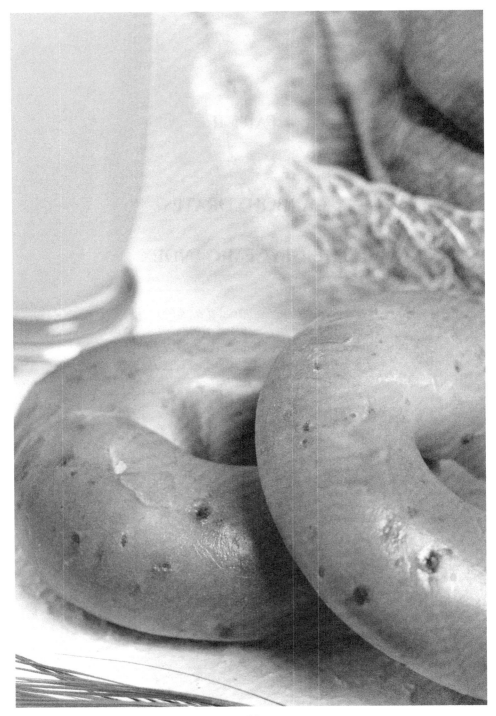

29

WHAT IS A CARB?

All this fear of carbohydrates, but I'm not even sure what a carb is.
Carbohydrates are either plant-based or fruit-based. They are found in starchy and non-starchy vegetables, bread, bagels, cereal, grains, sweets, pasta, fruit, milk, yogurt, and many other dairy products. Carbs can be real or man-made. Avoid man-made carbs.
Carbs are one of three fuel sources for the body. The other two are alcohol and fat. Carbs are the primary source of blood glucose and the preferred source of energy for the brain. However, the backup is ketone bodies that the liver extracts primarily from fatty acids in our body fat or diet. Low carb/higher fat will help the body produce ketones in the liver to be used as energy. They are a far superior energy source versus carbs.

Aren't there two specific types of carbs?
Yes. Carb are divided into simple or complex carbohydrates. Simple carbs include table sugar (sucrose), milk sugar (lactose), and fruit sugar (fructose). Simple carbs, those found in such food, as cookies, candy, sodas, white bread, most breakfast cereals, fruits, fruit juices, milk (more so, skim, low fat and fat free milk), etc., quickly affect the body, causing blood sugar levels to rise too high. This response causes insulin levels to spike, perpetuating carbohydrate cravings, fat storage, depression, and so forth.

Complex carbs, those found in whole grains and vegetables, though still made up of sugar molecules, are made up of longer, more complex chains. They're slower burning, slower to metabolize into energy, which means they do not affect blood sugar levels in such a dramatic manner. Either way, when you eat simple or complex carbohydrates, they are converted into glucose. This glucose is then either used immediately to supply energy to the body, or it's stored in the form of glycogen.

BEWARE: Liquid carbs, i.e., smoothies, fruit juice, etc., affect blood sugar levels far more dramatically than solid carbs. Avoid liquid carbs.

How does the body use carbs?
The brain uses glucose, a form of sugar, as its primary source of energy. The brain actually uses over 2/3 of the carbohydrates circulating in the bloodstream while you're resting. To maintain this high demand, the body continually takes carbohydrates and converts them into glucose. To reiterate, any carbohydrates that are not used right away by the body will be stored in the form of glycogen for later use. But if all of the glycogen stores are full, the extra glucose is converted into body fat. Another reason you must limit your carbohydrate intake, choose your carbs wisely, and increase your level of resistance training.

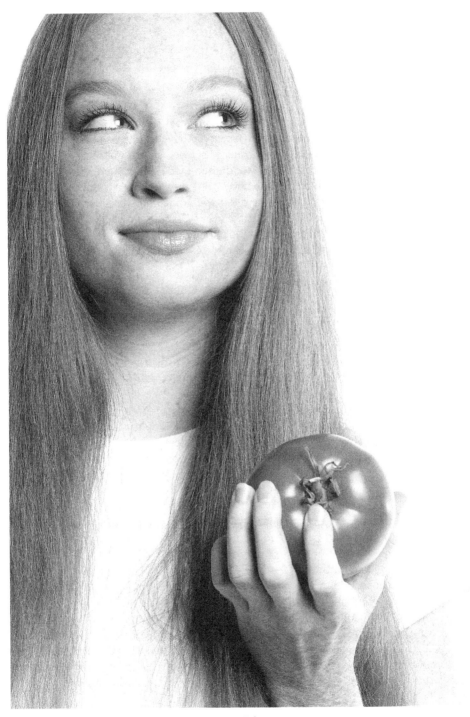

30

GOOD CARB? BAD CARB?
Which is it?

First and foremost, all carbs are not bad. The carbs you need to avoid are the highly refined, processed carbs such as breakfast cereals, pasta, candy, bread, rice, snack food, etc. In other words, *high glycemic carbs*. Unfortunately, one of the most popular, but equally unhealthy, carbs is shown in the previous chapter. And, yes, that would be bagels. And, again, your body converts both simple and complex carbs into sugar.

Bagels? I thought bagels were a healthy choice?
Sorry, bagels are one of the worst choices when it comes to carbs, for the mere fact that to get them to taste so moist and delicious, they're highly refined. Which means that as soon as you eat them, they turn into blood sugar, spiking insulin dramatically. If you insist on eating a bagel (which I hope you do not, because it's not a healthy food), you're better off eating a multi-grain bagel, though still excessively high in carbs, along with some sort of healthy fat and protein. Eggs, butter, avocado, turkey, cheese, etc., are all great choices, as this food will help lower the blood sugar response compared to eating just a plain bagel. And make sure you combine this food, never eating your carbs first, or alone, as you want to avoid spiking your insulin. I also recommend you eat your protein first, as it will signal your brain that food is coming and will, as a result, help control your appetite naturally.

Diets like Atkins make it seem like all carbs are evil. Are they?
All carbs are not bad. With regard to Atkins, he did not condemn all carbs. People often misinterpret his recommendations. It's primarily during the induction stage of his program that he asks you to seriously limits carbs. That meant eating only 20g of low GI, non-starchy carbs per day. His goal is to put the body into ketosis. The theory of ketosis is that, by depleting the body's glycogen stores, you force the body to use its stored body fat for fuel.

What is the glycemic index?
The glycemic index (GI) was created in the 1980s by a team of researchers. It is a guide for helping control diabetes. The GI is widely accepted in Canada, England, and Australia to help control not only diabetes, but also as an overall diet strategy. Just recently, the U.S. has come to realize the importance of this nutrition breakthrough. However, as great as I believe this system is, there's flaws in it, as well, because not all low glycemic carbs are healthy. Examples: Ice cream, pasta, Snickers bar, milk chocolate, etc.

How does it work?

The GI ranks, on a scale from 1–100, the speed at which carbs are converted into blood sugar. Pure glucose is the benchmark, with a rating of 100. Carbs that breakdown quickly during digestion have the highest GI value. This conversion triggers the rapid release of insulin. Insulin's primary role at this time is to protect the brain from this dangerous over-load of sugar.

Can you please explain it again?

All carbohydrates are recognized as sugar by the body, but they're ranked quite differ-ently based on how quickly they affect blood sugar levels. On this scale of 1–100, 1–54 is considered low GI. 55–70 is considered medium GI. 71–100 is considered high GI. Please note, this only measures quantity, *not quality*. For example: While white bread has a higher GI than a chocolate bar, the candy would also send your insulin levels soaring for hours. High levels of insulin, especially over long periods of time, are extremely harmful to your health. They can lead to insulin resistance, diabetes, and heart disease. Insulin is a hor-mone, and when it's elevated, it will upset every other hormone. Insulin also encourages the storage of body fat. Remember, insulin is the garage door opener to our fat cells.

Insulin actually opens fat cells?

Insulin stimulates the body's 30+ billion fat cell receptors and deposits carbohydrate energy directly into their interiors. This is how the body stores fat. With every meal, blood sugar levels rise. The key to maintaining a lean, healthy body is to keep your insulin levels stabilized. Therefore, please limit all such carbs, focusing on non-starchy, low GI carbs, as they cause the least amount of insulin production. Though the GI rating of carbs is what you need to concern yourself with most, it's not perfect either, as eating too many low GI carbs can equally trigger insulin. On the other hand, you can actually lower the GI rating of a high GI carb by eating a good quality fat and protein along with it.

Is this what all those "net carb/impact carb" products are referring to?

These products are merely subtracting the fiber from total carbs. But please do not fall for this deceptive marketing ploy. I agree some carbs are better than others, as well as carbs that affect blood sugar levels at different intensity, simple versus complex, but at the end of the day, I want to know how many *total carbs* I've eaten and the quality of those carbs. My bigger concern is that since the food industry has finally shifted from the all-consuming "fat free" movement, it has done a 180-degree turnaround to literally everything claiming to be LOW CARB. From low carb milk, low carb yogurt, to carb friendly cookies. Not to mention every restaurant advertisement is touting their low carb menus. Everyone has jumped on this bandwagon. This could all prove to be highly beneficial in the war against obesity, but only if the consumer really understands what low carb means. Unfortunately, this is rarely the case. I find it a fascinating study to watch people as they grocery shop. It's all-telling and rather frightening. It also confirms my fears about what this whole low carb/net carb movement is going to do to our obesity rate. Please allow me...

I was out shopping with Cookie, an adorable 10-year-old girl that I mentor. As we stood in the checkout line, I quietly observed the woman ahead of us. Her basket was filled with junk food. Oh, she had quite an assortment of goodies, ranging from several bags of sugar free candy, Keebler's Carb Sensible Chocolate-Chip Cookies, SnackWells CarbWell Fudge Brownie Cookies, sugar free cookies, low carb crackers, low carb chips, to a dozen low carb Hershey chocolate bars, which, by the way, were claiming a mere 2 net carbs. But hold on a minute! Do not be overly critical when judging this woman's choices. After all, I knew that, based on what she was buying, i.e., all LOW CARB and/or SUGAR FREE, she *believed* she was doing the right thing.

Sugar free cookies?
Ahhhh, a dream come true! Or, so you think.

You see, this woman clearly believed, that based on her items of choice, she was buying food that would keep her thin, or at least keep her from gaining any more weight. How terribly wrong, though. She's going to be in for a big and not so pleasant surprise as she starts to pack on the pounds. This disturbing scenario is a perfect example of most Americans' buying habits. Sorry to say, but most people tend to believe whatever food manufacturers claim on their labels. They assume they're being honest in their claims. This woman, and millions more just like her, will focus on buying all these bogus low carb, net/ impact carb and sugar free food, yet wonder why the hell they're getting heavier and more depressed than ever.

Are you starting to see why all this deceptive marketing is going to further fuel obesity, diabetes, heart disease, and cancer? Beware. This has quickly become the next multi-billion-dollar opportunity for food manufacturers. With the FDA and FTC setting few, if any regulations, a manufacturer can, in fact claim "low carb/sugar free" without any such proof. Without standards or regulations, how can one determine what is truly low carb or sugar free? This is just one of many reasons why I wrote this book: To help educate the consumer so they can hopefully make wiser and healthier choices.

Aren't the net carb claims found mostly on diet food and protein bars?
These claims are now found on all health bars, as well as everything from chips, crackers, cookies, milk, bagels, yogurt, cereal, to even ice cream. This is exactly why you need to seriously question the legitimacy of these claims. Compare "real carbohydrate" claims to these invented, processed carbs. Do you see them claiming on an avocado or a bag of mixed greens: "Only 3 Net Carbs!" No, of course not.

What about protein bars?
To reiterate, I'd like to believe the protein bar market was originally created to provide a healthy way for athletes to get extra protein. But due to the phenomenal success of this market, these quasi health, nutritional, and meal replacement bars have become nothing more than over-hyped, overpriced candy bars. Reading the various labels is proof enough. They're loaded with all kinds of additives, a ton of hidden sugars, HFCS, chocolate, fillers, etc. They are not a healthy choice, and they're definitely not a free food. Meaning: You

cannot eat them all day long and think they won't show up on your tummy. Among many things, they will most certainly perpetuate cravings.

So many overweight people, people who have never seen the inside of a gym, yet they're filling their grocery carts with these bars. I know darn well, though, based on the clever, million-dollar marketing strategy put forth by the manufacturers, the consumer is seduced into believing they're doing the right thing. Once again: Please, eat *real* food instead of these highly processed bars. (I must admit I eat a protein bar on a very rare occasion. But I also realize they are nothing more than a glorified candy bar with added protein.)

The power of branding. The power of manipulation.

I'd like to share the following, as it's a perfect example of just how easy it is to be fooled with product labels and their various claims, be it with regard to low carb, sugar free, or otherwise: A certain male celebrity recently launched an alternative to the standard, highly processed protein bar. It's a ready-to-eat, deliciously creamy, high protein pudding that comes in either milk chocolate or vanilla cream. Each individual 6.4 ounce can contains 20g of protein, a mere 1g of carbs, 2g of total fat, 0 trans fat, 330mg of potassium, 100 calories, 5mg of cholesterol, free of lactose, and 420mg of sodium.

My primary point here, though, is that they claim the pudding is SUGAR FREE. Now, as you have learned, nothing that sweet can be truly sugar free. If it's not naturally occurring sugar or they didn't physically add sugar on the front end, then how can they claim sugar free? Easy. They used sucralose, an artificial sweetener.

While I love the unique concept behind the very convenient packaging of a protein snack, my concern is with the sucralose they're using to sweeten the product. As mentioned earlier, sucralose is chemically altered and the subsequent health risks are numerous. This would have made for an excellent protein alternative to bars had they used stevia, in lieu of sucralose.

The ironic part of this story is that only days after reviewing this pudding, I saw a trainer in the gym eagerly devouring several of these protein puddings. All the while, he was raving to his client about how terrific it was, because "not only was it high in protein, but better yet, it was also *sugar free!"* The client was, of course, just as eager to go buy some. And as much as I wanted to say something, it wasn't my place. Unfortunately, as you can see, even most fitness experts aren't aware of the rules, and yes, trickery, behind the manufac- turers claims of their products being so-called "sugar free."

My suggestion would be that, first and foremost, manufacturers be held to the strictest of guidelines as to declaring what is truly in their food. Then, instead of the endless deceptive "sugar free, fat free, low carb, net carb" product claims, they should honestly, and accu- rately, state the "GI Rating" on all their products, as the GI is the critical factor in whether or not insulin is triggered. I believe this will, in fact, be the next big wave in product labeling. Will they be honest, though, is the real concern.

In closing this chapter, I simply had to add what I recently witnessed while Billy and I were training in a local gym. I saw the manager of this fitness chain come in and happily leave a large plate, *overflowing with bagel slices,* at the greeting desk. I couldn't believe she would do this. *Why would I be so shocked?* Because, as you know by now, bagels are one of the worst carbs for triggering insulin, and thus, causing the body to store fat. This high GI carb will also perpetuate cravings for more of the same. Yet here was the manager of this fitness facility eagerly supplying (and for free) this insulin-producing carb to her loyal members, members who were in her gym doing their best to lose weight, only for her to sabotage their efforts. If it wasn't so sad, I'd laugh. Nevertheless, either this woman was so completely unaware of this type of high GI carb and its subsequent affect on blood sugar levels, or she, in fact, knows the emotional attachment the bagel will have on her members, which will most definitely, on a subconscious level, have them coming back for more. I'd venture to guess she's not that aware, and instead, still pushing the low fat myth, which would also explain why she, herself, needed to lose 25 pounds.

One more example: A gym I trained at while in Utah, displayed huge signs introducing an exciting new workout program. They proudly offered the members FREE orange juice and bagels with the initial program launch. This was in addition to the dishes of chocolate found on nearly every counter as you walked through the lobby and locker rooms. Bagels? Juice? *Candy in a gym?* And all for FREE?! How generous, more so, how terribly disconcerting. Not forgetting the front desk people who I watched gorge on chocolate cake, bags of potato chips, and slurp on jumbo sodas, all while working.

Sorry, but there's no excuse for this. It would, though, help explain why nearly every trainer and employee was 25 to 100 pounds overweight. While I understand why so many people struggle with their weight, I find it disturbing that a "fitness" facility, whose goal is to supposedly get, and keep, their members healthy, would eagerly offer (and consume) such unhealthy food. Furthermore, where is the sense of company pride? Wouldn't they feel it's imperative to retain employees, especially their trainers, who'd show through their own bodies, what's possible by working out? Subsequently, to those who walk into this professed fitness facility, the usual motivating factor is, unfortunately, completely missing.

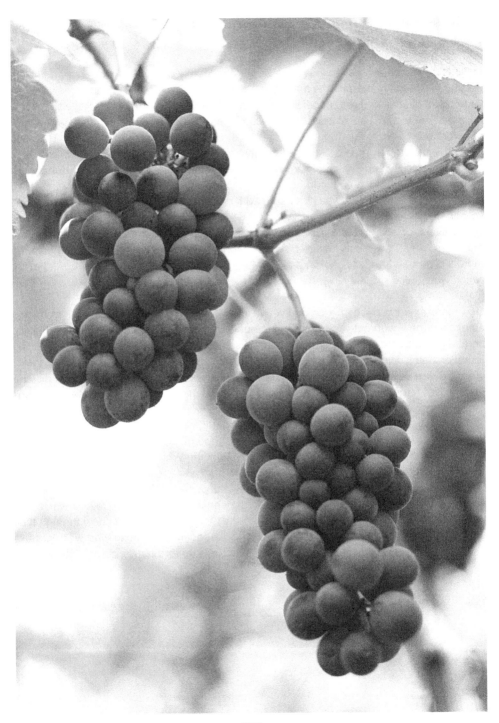

31

CRUCIAL CARBOHYDRATE FACTS

▶ Achieving optimum health is not just about eating low carb. It's also about eating higher fat. Your brain is 60% fat. It thrives on healthy fat and cholesterol.

▶ Simple carbs (fruit and candy) and complex carbs (vegetables and grains) are both broken down in the digestive system into one-sugar molecules.

▶ Simple carbohydrates consist of 1 to 2 linked sugar molecules. Complex carbohydrates consist of 3 and more linked sugar molecules.

▶ All carbohydrates, minus fiber, are recognized as "SUGAR" by the body.

▶ Fruit, though natural, is still a simple carbohydrate and high in fructose. Avoid eating fruit alone, or first. Never blend or break it down. Instead, eat it early day, combine it with a healthy fat and quality protein.

▶ Want to lose excess body fat effortlessly, lower BP, increase energy, look and feel decades younger, lower your trigs, stabilize cholesterol, alleviate depression and anxiety, ADD and insomnia, reduce risks of certain cancers, and more? Then please drink your water, keep your daily carbs to 20g and under, and eat 80g of healthy fat.

▶ Want to truly know what you're eating? Learn how to track your macros. (Best macro app: LOSE IT) These numbers will vary, but daily goals should be close to: CARBS 20g, FAT 80-110g, PROTEIN 60-90g / *20-30g per meal. We all have different health and fitness goals, so please eat accordingly. Note: Your body can only use a certain amount of protein per sitting; every 1.5 to 2 hours, hence, limiting to 20-30g.

▶ Carbohydrates are the only nutrient group that quickly converts into blood sugar.

▶ Unlike carbs, your body will let you know when you've eaten enough fat and protein.

▶ Liquid carbohydrates, i.e., milk, fruit juice, wine, smoothies, etc., are absorbed by the body much quicker than solids, which gives them a higher GI response.

▶ Never eat carbohydrates alone. Instead, combine them with a healthy (non-damaged) fat and quality protein so as to help lower the GI.

- Most glycogen is stored in the liver and in muscle cells. When these are saturated with glycogen, excess glucose, from carbs, will be converted to fat and stored as adipose tissue.

- Stop eating by 4-5p if you want to get leaner, quicker.

- Eat healthy carbs early day versus late, as it gives the body a chance to burn them off. I eat my carbs at breakfast and lunch. If I eat dinner; protein and fat only.

- Though pasta, cereal, and bread are considered to be complex carbs, they're highly refined man-made carbs. Avoid man-made carbs, as they require no digestion time, which means they quickly breakdown into blood sugar, thereby, affecting insulin levels dramatically.

- My favorite fruit? Avocado. They're rich in monounsaturated fat and polyphenols. Polyphenols are extremely important for gut health, and thus, overall health of the mind and body. I eat one or two every single day.

- I avoid most simple carbs/fruit due to the fructose. Plus, be it sugar from fruit or other-wise, sugar will cause cravings for more sugar and it can trigger my anxiety.

- Grapefruit and lemons are rich in citric acid, vitamin C and polyphenols. They are a low GI fruit. In addition to avocados, I eat them often, but always with a fat and protein.

- Starchy carbs (potatoes, rice, bread, pasta, etc.), will most often trigger insulin. I avoid starchy carbs. I have no desire to eat them, because my serotonin levels are stable.

- Avoid eating carbs alone. Always combine with fat and/or protein.

- Even though some carbs may be considered low GI, it may, nevertheless, still be high in useless carbs, sugar, etc.

- You can eat more of low GI carbs, or less of high GI carbs, and still achieve the same blood sugar levels.

- Avoid nightshade vegetables: bell peppers, tomatoes, eggplant, potatoes, hot peppers, tomatillos and goji berries. They contain lectins. They're known as anti-nutrients.

- When considering insulin levels, it's not only the GI you should be concerned with, but also the amount, and quality, of all carbohydrates consumed.

- When it comes to eating carbs, quality, quantity, and time of day eaten are crucial to factors to remember.

▶ Just because the crackers, pizza, chips, etc., are gluten free, it doesn't mean they're a healthy choice. Avoid gluten, yes, but also understand what you're eating.

▶ With regard to fruit, avocado, olives, grapefruit and strawberries have the lowest GI.

▶ Want antioxidants? Sure, we all do. Pecans are much higher in antioxidants than blueberries — and without the fruit sugar. Pecans are packed with vitamin A, vitamin E, folic acid, calcium, magnesium, phosphorus, potassium, several B vitamins and zinc. It only takes about an ounce (about 8 pecans) to get these nutritional and antioxidant benefits.

▶ In summary, please choose your food with the greatest of care, be it carbs, fat, and/or protein. And, remember, your gut is like the Amazon rainforest. Your body contains trillions of bacteria, viruses, and fungi. They're known as the microbiome. The gut microbiome refers to all of the microbes in the intestines, which act like another organ. They're vital for optimum health. While some bacteria are associated with disease, others are extremely important for the immune system, heart, weight, and countless other aspects of our health. So, please, feed your gut with the greatest of care. I also recommend Ora organic prebiotic/probiotic powder. However, all the supplements in the world will not matter, if your food and/or lifestyle choices are unhealthy.

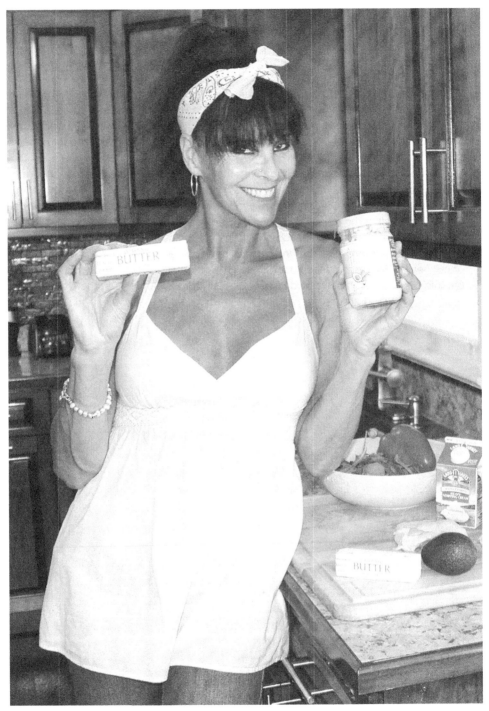

32

MY PERSONAL MEALS THAT WILL HELP YOU
Lose body fat, improve lipids,
alleviate depression, increase energy—and more

It was imperative that I dedicate a chapter to the food I eat, as well as how my clients achieve extraordinary success. First rule; buy real food, food that is fresh, raw ingredients, never pre-packaged, and mostly, organically grown. Be aware that the FDA does not have any set guidelines when it comes to food manufacturers who make these claims. I also make sure I do not buy the things I know I shouldn't eat. There is absolutely no effort for me to eat this way, as long as I maintain my serotonin. I <u>never</u> feel deprived.

Next, you want your body burning body fat and the fat you eat, not carbs. To achieve this, please keep your low GI carbs to around 20g daily—and no alcohol or wine. This forces your body from burning all those useless carbs as energy, to burning fat. Fat is the far superior fuel source. You need fat to burn fat. The brain also thrives on fat.

The following foods are what work best for me, and my clients, be it physically, mentally, and emotionally. They're clean. Simple. Healthy. When you eat, please stop and ask yourself: *"Will this food nourish my mind and body, or, will it create disease?"*

When transitioning to this healthy way of eating, to help avoid the "carb flu," please use quality sea salt in your water daily. Use it thereafter, as it's vital to good health.

MACROS: Fat, carbohydrates, and protein are called macronutrients. Food comes with a blend of these macronutrients.

▶ **PRIMARY PROTEIN OPTIONS w/ FAT:** Organic eggs, salmon, sardines, mackerel, anchovies, catfish, cod liver, shrimp, lobster, scallops, skipjack tuna (AVOID ahi and albacore due to high mercury), chicken, turkey, ribeye, beef liver, lamb, "Naked Egg" brand egg white protein powder

▶ **PRIMARY FAT OPTIONS w/ PROTEIN:** Goat, sheep, ricotta, mozzarella, Brie, Muenster, Havarti, Parmesan, Folio cheese wraps, avocado, olives, full fat cottage cheese, lactose free sour cream, cream cheese, (*Fresh/white cheese is healthiest. Limit aged/yellow. Avoid shredded cheese due to unhealthy fillers: cellulose, potato starch, corn starch, etc.)

▶ **CLEAN FAT OPTIONS:** ("clean" basically means no other macros) EVOO (CA Olive Ranch brand), ghee, avocado oil (AO), walnut oil, butter, MCT oil, avocado oil mayo (Primal Kitchen brand), unrefined coconut oil, heavy whipping cream (HWC)

▶ **PRIMARY CARB OPTIONS:** Arugula, spinach, celery, hearts of palm, bok choy, cilantro, cauliflower, mashed cauliflower, marinated artichoke hearts, mushrooms, capers, asparagus, angel
hair coleslaw, macadamias, pecans, walnuts, chia & sunflower seeds
MY FAVORITE LOW GI FRUIT OPTIONS: Avocado, olives, zucchini, cucumber, lemon, grapefruit

▶ **HERBS/SPICES:** Cilantro, dill, tarragon, curry, turmeric, pepper, Redmond Real Sea Salt (SS)
▶ **BEVERAGES**: Unsweetened almond/coconut milk, caffeine free herbal tea
▶ **NATURAL SWEETENER:** Stevia (SweetLeaf brand)
▶ **HEALTHY TREATS:** FAT BOMBS: 1 stick butter, half a tsp unsweetened cacao powder, 1/4-c
unrefined coconut oil, 1/4-c chopped hazelnuts, English toffee stevia, mix, simmer ingredients over
low heat until melted. Pour into glass dish. Freeze 20 minutes. Delicious!
DARK CHOCOLATE: 2 pieces 98% cocoa plain or w/ 1/4-c full fat ricotta cheese
FULL FAT RICOTTA: 1/4-c w/ 1/8-c pecans, dash cinnamon

If you're not used to eating fat, start slowly: 1 tbsp clean fat per meal, working up to two tbsp
The body can only absorb 25-30g protein per meal/sitting: every 1.5 to 2 hrs

BREAKFAST & LUNCH OPTIONS: (Aim for 20-30g of protein per breakfast and lunch)
Note: Amount of protein per oz in primary source will vary, i.e., chicken vs fish, lamb, beef, etc.)
▶ Crustless quiche: 3 eggs, 2 tbsp butter, 1/4-c HWC, 1 oz chicken, 1-c oooked mushrooms
▶ Romaine lettuce wraps: 3 oz shrimp, 1 tbsp ghee, 1/4-c avocado, 1 tbsp EVOO, cilantro
▶ Chicken thigh, 4 oz, sautéed in 2 tbsp ghee, 3 stalks hearts of palm, 1 oz mozzarella, SS
▶ Arugula 1-c, 1 oz goat cheese, 1 HB egg, 3 oz salmon, 1 tbsp EVOO, 6 Kalamata olives,
1 tbsp avocado mayo, 1/4-c sunflower seeds, pepper, lemon
▶ Cold seafood stack: 4 oz diced shrimp, crab, 1/2 grapefruit, cilantro, lime, 2 tbsp EVOO
▶ Salmon, 4 oz, dill, 1 tbsp ghee, lemon, 1-c asparagus, SS, 1 tbsp butter, 1 oz sheep cheese
▶ 3 eggs, 1 tbsp ghee, 1/4-c pecans, 1/2-c full fat cottage cheese, 1 tbsp EVOO
▶ Lamb chop, 3 oz, 1 tbsp butter, 2-c wilted bok choy, pepper, 1 tbsp avocado mayo
▶ Crab cake w/ real crab, 1 tbsp butter, lemon, 1-c cooked baby portobellos, 1 tbsp ghee
▶ Skipjack tuna, 4 oz, 1 tsp capers, 2 diced anchovies, lemon, 1 tbsp EVOO, 1/2 grapefruit
▶ Cod liver, 3 oz, 2 chopped HB eggs, w/ 1/2-c diced cucumber, 2 tbsp sour cream
▶ 3 HB eggs, cilantro, 1 oz Parmesan, 2 tbsp EVOO, 2-c arugula, 1/4-c sunflower seeds
▶ Sardines, 3 oz, 1/2-c artichoke hearts, 1/4-c pecans, 1 oz fresh Parmesan
▶ Chicken breast, 4 oz, 1 tbsp EVOO, 2-c wilted arugula, 1 tbsp EVOO, 1/4-c walnuts
▶ Broiled halibut, 3 oz, 1 tbsp butter, lemon, sea salt, 1-c zucchini, 1 tbsp sour cream, SS
▶ Turkey patty, 3 oz, 1 tbsp ghee, 2-c bok choy, 1 oz sheep cheese, 1 tbsp butter, parsley, lime
▶ Omelet: 3 eggs whipped, 1 tbsp butter, 2-c wilted spinach, top w/ 1/4-c ricotta cheese
▶ Scallops, 4 oz, lemon, 1 tbsp ghee, 2-c leafy greens, 1/4-c kalamata olives, 2 oz sheep cheese
▶ Baked catfish, 3 oz, 1 tbsp butter, 1-c mashed cauliflower, pepper, 1 tbsp AO, SS
▶ Whole avocado, 1/2-c full fat cottage chese, top w/ 4 oz sardines
▶ Ribeye steak, 4 oz, 1 tbsp butter, 1-c asparagus, 1 tbsp EVOO, pepper, SS
▶ Beef liver, 4 oz, 2-c bok choy, sautéed in 2 tbsp butter, pepper
▶ Fresh lobster, 4 oz, 6 diced greek olives, over 2-c arugula, 2 tbsp EVOO, pepper, lime, SS

DINNER OPTIONS: (Aim for 20g of protein)
▶ 2 scoops Naked Egg protein powder, 8 oz UNSW coconut milk, nutmeg, stevia, 1/4-c HWC
▶ Sauté 3 oz mackerel, 1-c wilted arugula, lemon, hot sauce, w/ 1 tbsp ghee
▶ Catfish, 3 oz, 1 tbsp ghee, lemon, 2 tsp capers, 1 tbsp spicy avocado mayo
▶ Sardines, 3 oz, sautéed in 1 tbsp butter, capers, lemon, over 1-c wilted kale, 1 tbsp EVOO
▶ Shrimp 8, 1 tbsp EVOO, 1/4-c black olives, garlic, cilantro, 2 tbsp sour cream
▶ Chicken thigh, 3 oz, 1 tbsp ghee, 1-c cooked mushrooms, 1/4-c ricotta cheese over thigh
▶ Folio cheese wrap, 1 tbsp butter, 3 oz ground turkey, 1/2 tbsp avocado mayo, SS
▶ Romaine wedge, top w/ 3 oz chicken breast, 1 tbsp butter, 1/2-c sauteed mushrooms, broil, SS
▶ Broiled scallops, 3 oz, 1 tbsp coconut oil, capers, 2-c wilted spinach, lemon, 1 oz sheep cheese
▶ Salmon bites (6), 1 tbsp ghee, 1/2-c full fat cottage cheese, 2 tbsp sour cream
▶ Turkey patty, 3 oz, 1 tbsp ghee, garlic, 1 oz Swiss, 2-c wilted bok choy, SS

TWO MEALS PER DAY / INTERMITTENT FASTING:
The latest studies show that eating just two meals a day, with intermittent fasting (IF), works great for weight loss, overall health, longevity, autophagy, etc. Start with the 18:6 split. (Eat two healthy meals between 11am and 5pm. Fast from 5pm to 11am. I eat two meals a day; large breakfast and late lunch. My clients either do IF with a large breakfast and lunch, or they eat two smaller meals, with a light dinner no later than 5p.

Want to get lean quickly, without tracking macros? Please follow these basic guidelines:
FAT: 2 tbsp clean fat at breakfast, lunch, and dinner (AO, ghee, EVOO, mayo, butter, etc.)
PROTEIN: 20-30g protein per meal
CARBS: Up to 20g daily. Low GI, non-starchy carbs, eaten mostly at breakfast and lunch
* I eat very few carbs. I eat mostly avocados, pecans, and olives

Everyone's body is different. Learn to listen to your body. Keep your serotonin balanced. My meals, however, will get you close to 80-100g fat, 60-90g protein, with carbs 20g and under, per day. Your goals are to reduce your body fat, trigs, and waist circumference so as to reduce the risks for various diseases: **Women:** waist < 30", BF 20-24%, trigs 40-60. **Men:** waist < 35", BF 14-17%, trigs 40-60.

TIPS: Eat largest meals early day. If you eat dinner, eat light and no later than 5p. Avoid triggering insulin. Read all labels. Water: drink 90 to 100 oz—or until your urine is light yellow. Add quality electrolytes to your water. Use sea salt daily. Get 7-9 hours of quality sleep. Take the 5 faithfully. Go to bed a bit hungry. Wake up leaner. Eat healthy. Repeat cycle. You have to be a bit hungry to change the body. For those who don't want to track macros and/or have stalled in their weight loss, try intermittent fasting. No matter what theory you choose, I recommend clean, healthy food. Low carb/higher fat/medium protein is the healthiest, most rewarding way of eating, and with too many exceptional health benefits to mention. Please, start now. Don't wait another minute.

WARNING: Limit seafood to 2-3 times per week due to mercury and other toxins.

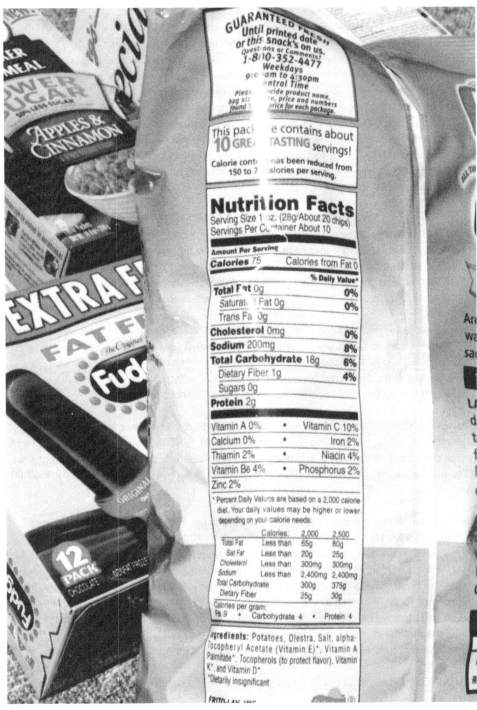

33

HOW TO READ A NUTRITION FACTS LABEL
Don't be fooled. Know what you're eating.

With so much deception, how will I ever really know what I'm eating?
As we discussed earlier, food and beverage manufacturers are required to provide certain nutrition facts on their products. This information has, unfortunately, proven to be far less than truthful, you still need to read the label to get an idea of what you're eating. Then learn to listen to your body. If something is sweet, ask *why.* If you feel a sugar/adrenaline rush after eating something, ask *why.* If you suddenly feel thirsty, read the label again and look for the amount of sodium. If you feel bloated, ask *why*. If you unexpectedly feel agitated, ask *why.* Read and reread food labels until you really begin to understand <u>how</u> and <u>why</u> food/beverages play such a critical role in your physical, emotional, and mental health.

As hard as I try, why is it so difficult to get through a grocery store without buying junk food? I can't seem to resist.
You're not alone, as it is a well-known fact grocery stores spend a great deal of time and money displaying their assorted food and beverages in a very precise and manipulative manner. They strategically place processed/high GI carbs at the front of the store and center aisles, while R-E-A-L food, i.e., seafood, meat, vegetables, etc., are on the outside aisles and in the rear of the store. Assorted chips, cookies, alcohol, flavored drinks, candy, bagels, etc., take front and center, placed at the beginning of each aisle. Don't forget, every checkout line is loaded with candy and other junk food. Well, understand this: It is not a coincidence. THIS IS ALL FOR A REASON. Those in charge know this food is an impulse item, a trigger food. They also know this food is highly *addictive.* Their motive: Sell this junk with no regard for our health. It is, once again, all about profits. This food perpetuates cravings, contributing to excessive fat gain, diabetes, depression, heart disease, cancer, etc. Beware of these marketing tactics.

Excuse me? You say candy doesn't tempt you? That's great to know. But how about this: The latest marketing ploy by grocery stores is having warm, wonderfully fresh baked bread placed on huge racks right at the entrance of every checkout line. This bread is so fresh, the steam is literally rising from it. So, as you patiently wait in line, trying to avoid the many other temptations placed before you, the smell of this bread is an even bigger tease. I ask you: *How many people can ignore this temptation?* How many people, who had no desire for bread, end up grabbing a loaf, based solely on this clever manipulation? If the bread isn't tempting enough, the stores are also now placing racks of Krispy Kreme donuts at the beginning of the aisles. I am simply amazed at the lengths the grocery stores go to control their unsuspecting customers. Again, buyer beware.

However, hold on a second. That's not all. The most recent marketing ploy by certain grocery stores is to have food on the actual turn aisle, at the end of where your groceries are bagged. It's not just any food, either. Oh, no, definitely not. It's only the food that the store knows are addictive, food such as cereal, candy, soda, chips, etc. The first time I saw this, I had to laugh. I mean, come on, *where does it end?* You've done your best to get through their manipulative aisles, you've succeeded in ignoring their attempts to seduce you with the endless rows of candy, fresh baked bread, and sinfully sweet smelling donuts, only to have them, at the checkout line, once again, so brazenly tempt and tease you with another bunch of sugar-laden, high GI carbs while you're trying to pay for your groceries. Worse yet, it doesn't stop there. If you're able to ignore whatever the chosen item is on display, an item that is literally shoved in your face, the cashier actually asks you if you'd like to purchase it. (And you better believe they will ask, as I was recently told by a cashier that they get penalized if they don't. Three points? They're fired. Whoa! Talk about corporate priorities.) The real concern, though, is: How many people will be able to refrain from this shrewd manipulation and endless temptation? Not many, I'm afraid.

Now that you are hopefully better informed as to these tactics, you will next need to know how to read, to interpret a food label. The following is the order in which I, personally, read a label. This will determine what I buy and, subsequently, put into my body. Nevertheless, before I even begin to read the label, and depending on the food source, I will check to see if the food is organically grown, range-free, hormone/antibiotic-free. You must also keep in mind that the FDA does not enforce the law that says all the ingredients in packaged/processed food must be listed. These are, of course, the hidden ingredients that food manufacturers <u>don't</u> what us to know about. These are the very ingredients that these companies sneak into our food, ingredients that further ensure we get addicted, coming back for more, and all the while make us fat, depressed, and sicker than ever. With that in mind, the following is the order in which I review nutrition facts and ingredient labels:

1) Ingredients:
I first look to see what the product is made of. This is where you'll find exactly what ingredients are in the product. This will let me know if I even want to buy this particular item. This section will list everything from the primary ingredient source (ranging from chicken, pork, beef, cheese, to flour, grains, starch, caffeine, hydrogenated fats, etc.) You'll also find additives, colorings, and the many hidden sugars, alternative sweeteners, and artificial sweeteners, such as aspartame, sucralose, acesulfame-K, HFCS, sugar alcohols, molasses, glycerine, etc., in this section. To reiterate, there is an exact science behind how these ingredients are listed. The ones listed first are the ones in *heaviest* concentrations, and so forth down the line. Please read this list with great consideration. And, if you can't pronounce the names of the ingredients, avoid that product.

2) Total Carbohydrate:

This is the most important one. The number shown is based on a single serving. I look to see how many grams are in each serving. Although complex and simple carbs affect the blood sugar levels at different rates, <u>all carbs, minus fiber, breakdown into sugar once consumed</u>. Consequently, I focus on the <u>total</u> number of carbs versus net carbs or amount of sugar. Per serving I prefer 0-7g. It's also important to note that I'm choosing healthy low GI, non-starchy carbs, not processed/refined/simple carbs. It's effortless to eat this way, because I maintain my serotonin, which controls cravings and appetite. My total carbs per day are under 20g. This works for me, based on my body type, goals, level of exercise, muscle mass, metabolic rate, and age. My primary source of carbs: arugula, celery, asparagus, cucumbers, mushrooms and avocado. The insulin response is bare minimum. I stay much leaner, healthier, *and far less anxious*, when I keep my carbs healthy, and to a minimum.

3) Serving Size:

Keep in mind that nutrition facts are based on a single serving size. This data is then broken down into precise categories. The total numbers shown reflect only that one serving size. Example: A small bag of chips may easily have 2 servings per bag. As a result, if you were to eat the entire bag, you'd have to double all the numbers shown to get the TOTAL number of carbs, sugar, sodium, fat, etc. Another example is a particular brand of protein powder. On their front label, they claim in huge letters: *"46g of PROTEIN"* Not quite. But you'd have to read the nutrition facts label to see that it would take 3 large scoops to actually get those 46g. *Deceptive marketing?* Not really. Misleading is more like it. Manufacturers realize that most consumers only read the front of the label, believing whatever the label claims. Compared to many of the other protein powders, 46g is huge. Hence, you buy it, naturally thinking you're getting more for your money. However, unless you read the serving size, you won't realize it takes twice, maybe three times, the amount of product to get that amount.

4) Net Carbs/Impact Carbs:

I ignore this number. It's not even regulated. Once again, while carbs certainly affect blood sugar levels differently, some burning slower and longer than others, there is no accurate way to measure this claim. Without any FDA regulations, as to what truly determines low carb or net/impact carbs, *consumer beware*. Focus on eating healthy non-starchy, low GI carbs, combining them with healthy fat and protein, and then account for the <u>total</u> number of carbs, not just their erratic claims of only net carbs/impact carbs. As I stated earlier, this is merely another deceitful marketing practice being imposed on the far too trusting consumer. My concern is how many (total) carbs they're claiming. Even that is often inaccurate. And, because of the deception, I merely look at what they claim for total carbs. I also pay very close attention to the ingredient list and order in which the ingredients are listed. All of this information combined, will give me a much better idea of what is in a particular product. (Food/beverage manufacturers should be required to declare the "GI Rating" of all their products. This would help consumers make far healthier choices.)

5) Sugars:

Though all carbs (minus the fiber) listed under Total Carbohydrate will "turn into sugar" once consumed, I still look at the amount of sugar the product is claiming to have. Keep in mind, the amount of sugar a product claims does <u>not</u> distinguish between sugars that are naturally occurring and those that are refined or artificial. I try to avoid all types of sugar and sweeteners, but it's nearly impossible. I do my best to limit what they "claim is sugar" to 0–3g per serving.

WARNING:

"No Sugar Added" or "Sugar Free" only means that the manufacturer didn't actually add sugar on the front end when making this product. Please, please, please, do not fall for this marketing ploy. It does not account for the carbs that will turn into sugar once they are consumed. It does not account for the sugars found naturally in the product. Nor does it account for alternative/artificial sweeteners, i.e., aspartame, sucralose, maltodextrin, neotame, maltitol, etc., that they may use to sweeten this alleged "SUGAR FREE" product. This is just another example of clever and misleading marketing tactics.

Example: Smucker's Sugar Free Jam. How can jam, which is made from fruit, possibly be sugar free? Easy. It's not. It's made from fruit, which contains fructose, i.e., fruit sugar. Because Smucker's did not physically add sugar to this product, nor do they have to account for the naturally occurring sugar, they can legally make this "sugar free" claim. Even more disturbing is when I read the ingredient panel. I was stunned to see they use ASPARTAME in their alleged wholesome food.

Another example: How can a package of cookies claim to be sugar free? Again, the manufacturer either did not physically add sugar on the front end or they used artificial sweeteners. Either way, once consumed, the body will recognize the exorbitant amount of high GI carbs in these cookies, as S-U-G-A-R.

6) Other Carbohydrate/Sugar Alcohols:

Beware. These items are listed below the area where you would normally look for carbs, sugar, protein, etc. Go to the bottom. Read the fine print. This category is relatively new and found only on professed carb-friendly food. To be honest, I have no idea what "Other Carbohydrate" are. It seems to be merely another marketing attempt to hide additional sugars, at the same time, hoping we get addicted to their food. After all, it's the sugar that makes things taste so good and keeps us coming back for more.

Sugar Alcohols: Food manufacturers claim they don't affect blood sugar levels. Many believe otherwise, as it's still a form of sugar. Nonetheless, sugar alcohols perpetuate cravings. To reiterate, they also play havoc on the digestive system, causing flatulence (gas) and diarrhea. Make sure you read the fine print. Avoid sugar alcohols.

7) Dietary Fiber:

Dietary fibers are indigestible (complex) carbs that pass through the intestinal tract without being absorbed. This is because the bacteria present in the digestive system lacks the enzymes required to breakdown the fiber. The fiber content means these particular carbs are slower burning and much slower to affect blood sugar levels. Experts claim you can subtract the amount of fiber from the total amount of carbs to get the "true" number of carbs. While this is true, with all the marketing deception regarding carbs, I don't believe most of what I read. So, I pick my carbs with great care. If you eat too many carbs and/or the wrong carbs, the body will prioritize them, and the cycle will repeat: You'll be burning glucose and glycogen for energy—while the excess will get stored, as body fat.

8) Protein:

Any protein noted is a plus, as long as it's a clean source. If it's a primary protein source, i.e., salmon, turkey, liver, chicken, etc., I like to see a range of 20-25g per serving. I eat a total of 20-30g per meal. My protein intake is based on my goals and LBM (lean body mass). Your protein needs will vary depending on your LBM, male or female, and whether or not you want to build muscle, lose weight, and how many times a day you eat. In order for muscle to grow, which plays a vital role in getting lean, you need to consume *more* protein than you utilize. As your weight and fitness goals change, so will your protein needs.

9) Total Fat:

Because of the type of food I buy, I never look at the fat. The higher the healthy fat, the better. I eat about 80-100g per day. Avoid trans fat. Saturated, polyunsaturated, and monounsaturated fats are all needed for a healthy body and mind. Perfect examples of saturated fat; butter, cheese, eggs, sour cream, avocado oil mayo, chicken and turkey fat. Excellent sources of monounsaturated fat are found in the following oils; olive, almond, and hazelnut. The following oils are wonderful sources of polyunsaturated fat; primrose, herring, salmon, and sardines. I get most of my fat from avocado, olives, sour cream, butter, EVOO, mackerel, avocado oil mayo, eggs, cheese, HWC, salmon, cod liver, anchovies and sardines. I eat 2-3 healthy fats with every meal. Please avoid seed oils.

I realize far too many people are still scared of eating fat, especially saturated fat. But you need to know there's a huge difference between eating the above fat versus the damaged fat you find in french fries, fried onion rings, donuts, pastries, etc. The body *needs* fat to rebuild bones, hair, hormones, cells, enzymes, muscles, and neurotransmitters. To reiterate, eating *healthy, non-damaged* fat does NOT make you fat, because it doesn't trigger insulin. So please, EAT FAT, but choose them wisely.

WARNING: Fat Free/Low Fat:

Avoid all food that makes this claim, as they are loaded with sugar, HFCS, corn syrup, etc. If this food isn't loaded with sugar, the fat free snack food often contain olestra, an indigestible fat substitute that causes serious side effects. BEWARE.

10) Sodium:

Sodium is needed to help control body fluids, maintain normal blood pressure, nerve, and muscle activity. However, if you're eating based on the typical American diet, which is filled with junk carbs, processed food, etc., please limit your sodium to 350mg per serving. Too much sodium, *without the other vital minerals found in a high quality sea salt,* can lead to hypertension, osteoporosis, kidney stones, stomach cancer, and other health risks. At bare minimum, too much sodium will make you extra thirsty and retain water, i.e., bloated. To remedy; drink water, flush your system, and move on. Then do your best to avoid junk carbs and processed food. I highly recommend Redmond Real Sea Salt, along with a low carb/higher fat diet. I use it often. Range 2,000mg to 4,000mg daily.

11) Calories:
When reading a nutrition label the only thing I never look at is calories. Why? Because calories are not created equal. EXAMPLE: 250 calories in a smoothie are entirely different than 250 calories in a chicken thigh. I, do, however, track my macros. I make sure I'm within a certain range on those. (This is also what I teach my clients.) But when I review a nutrition facts label, I'm looking at the protein, fat and carbs, among other factors, but I never look, nor care about, what they claim the calories are. Again, I eat approximately 80-100g of fat daily, which are CALORIE DENSE, yet my body fat remains low at just 13% and I'm disease free. Calories are, again, not created equal.

12) Calories from Fat:
Same applies here, as above. I do not count calories from fat. I eat an abundance of healthy fat. This is, once again, because of the food I choose, along with keeping my serotonin maintained.

13) Cholesterol:
I want cholesterol in my food, because we need to eat cholesterol to shut down our body's internal clock from producing its own. If you don't, your body will make cholesterol from the high GI carbs you eat. This will drive up your LDL. Therefore, you need to eat healthy cholesterol with every meal, which can be found in food, such as eggs, shellfish, cheese, poultry, fish, organ meat, and butter. This is absolutely factual, because as I mentioned earlier, I eat plenty of fresh cheese, poultry, shellfish, four sticks of butter and two dozen eggs every week, and my cholesterol panels are exceptional. My focus with respect to a healthy cholesterol panel is to avoid any insulin-producing carbs, beverages and/or substances. Maintaining your serotonin will help you do this effortlessly. Beyond that, having a healthy heart comes from living a healthy lifestyle.

14) Vitamins, Minerals, and Other Information:
This lists the various vitamins, minerals, and nutrients in the food and their daily percent values. It's best to try to average daily 100% DV for vitamins A, C, calcium, fiber, and iron. (To be honest, based on the healthy food I eat, I never read this.)

▶ *Sugar Free*: The product has to contain less than 1/2g of sugar per serving. However, and I cannot say this enough: Sugar free only means that the manufacturers did not physically add sugar on the front end. It does not account for the carbs that will *turn into* sugar once consumed. Nor does it account for the sugars found naturally in the product. And it definitely does not account for the harmful artificial sweeteners used.

❱ *Gluten Free:* This only means that the product is without gluten. It does not mean the food is a healthy choice, i.e., gluten free pizza, crackers, chips, bread, etc.

❱ *Reduced Sugar:* 25% or less sugar per serving than the principle food

❱ *Calorie Free/No Calories:* Contains less than 5 calories per serving

❱ *Low Calorie:* Contains 1/3 the calories of the original version or a similar product

❱ *Lite:* Contains 1/3 the calories or 1/2 the fat per serving of the original version

❱ *Fat Free/No Fat:* Must contain less than 1/2g of fat per serving

❱ *Reduced Fat/Lower Fat:* 25% or less fat per serving than the principle food

❱ *Low Fat:* Contains less than 3g of fat per serving

❱ *No Preservatives Added:* May contain *natural* preservatives, but none "added"

❱ *No Preservatives:* Contains no preservatives, chemical or natural

❱ *Low Sodium:* Contains less than 140mg of sodium per serving

❱ *No Salt/Salt Free:* Contains less than 5mg of sodium per serving

❱ *Good Source of Fiber*: 2.5g to 5g per serving

❱ *More/Added Fiber:* Contains 2.5g or more fiber per serving than the principle food

❱ *High Fiber:* 5g or more fiber per serving

Definitions:
g = gram
mg = milligram
mcg = microgram
tsp = teaspoon
tbsp = tablespoon
1 serving size = the amount of food that can, in theory, fit in the palm of your hand

IN CLOSING THIS CHAPTER:
Just because the Nutrition Facts Label may claim
zero sugar and/or zero carbs,
it does not mean that food is a healthy choice.
There's so much more to it than that.
Learn how to truly comprehend
the Nutrition Facts and Ingredient Labels.
This will help ensure your success in getting lean and healthy.

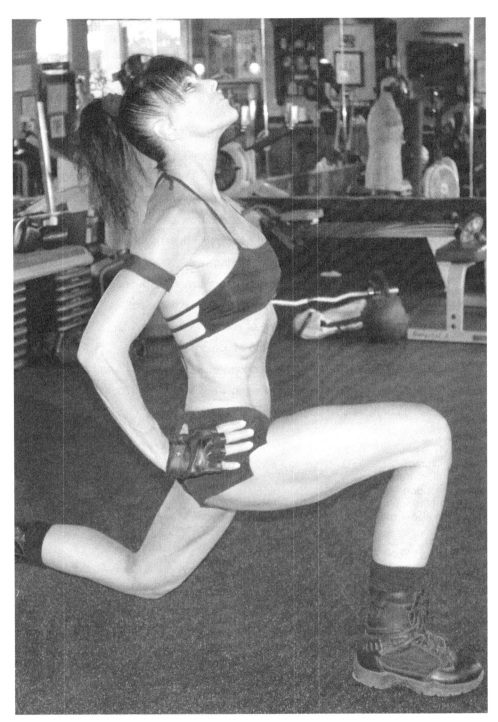

Age 57

34

A SUMMARY OF HEALTH TIPS
THAT WILL HELP YOU ACHIEVE
OPTIMUM HEALTH

I hope you realize I've tried to share this information with you in an easy-to-understand type of dialogue. (It's also based on actual conversations with various clients.) Nothing is worse, though, than when you finally get motivated to improve your health and you go out and buy the latest diet/health/fitness books, only to discover that far too often these books are filled with over-the-top medical jargon that even those individuals in the health industry can't comprehend. I promise that if you read this book, *until you really get it,* your life will forever be changed. Guaranteed!

Keeping that in mind, I wanted to summarize some of the health facts you just read about. Hopefully, this list will help you understand it all even more than you already do.

▶ 98% of all attempts to lose weight will inevitably fail, unless you're able to properly maintain serotonin, a major neurotransmitter.

▶ Serotonin is depleted by everything from stress, alcohol, sugar, high GI carbs, lack of deep restorative sleep, processed/refined food, artificial sweeteners, prescription, non-prescription, and street drugs, nicotine, caffeine, ephedrine, dieting (especially low fat dieting), lack of exercise, etc.

▶ People often feel as if they are addicted to certain carbs, because they increase the production of serotonin, a wonderful, mood-altering brain chemical.

▶ When serotonin is depleted, our brain will force us on a *subconscious* level toward high GI carbs. Its primary goal is to both boost serotonin and provide the quickest fuel to the brain. Both of which are achieved by consuming these high GI carbs. To boost serotonin in this manner, however, insulin must first be triggered.

▶ Insulin is the hormone that opens fat cells. Hence, causing the body to store fat.

▶ A diet high in processed/high GI carbs = high insulin levels/low serotonin levels.

▶ A diet high in sugar = high insulin levels/low serotonin levels.

▶ A diet high in caffeine/stimulants = high insulin levels/low serotonin levels.

▶ High insulin levels = high body fat storage ratio, water retention, abnormal thyroid and hormone function, harmful cholesterol profile, plaquing of the arteries, high blood pressure, increased risks of cancer, heart disease, stroke, diabetes, etc.

▶ Low serotonin = high GI carb/sugar cravings, bulimia, obesity, rage, sudden outbursts, mood swings, ADD/ADHD, agitation, depression, anxiety, panic attacks, PMS, insomnia, alcoholism, headaches, migraines, chronic body pain, lethargy, decreased libido, OCD, irritable bowel syndrome, memory loss, schizophrenia, suicidal behavior, etc.

▶ Controlling cravings = less insulin.

▶ Less insulin = less body fat stored, more body fat utilized as fuel.

▶ Less insulin = lowering risks for obesity, diabetes, high blood pressure, heart attack, stroke, certain cancers, etc.

▶ Less insulin = healthier cholesterol and thyroid panels.

▶ Higher body fat = less lean muscle mass (plus, higher triglycerides and increased risks for diabetes, heart disease, certain cancers, stroke, high blood pressure, etc.)

▶ Less lean muscle mass = slower metabolism/lower BMR, less calories/fat burned.

▶ More lean muscle mass = faster, more effective metabolism/higher BMR. *Why?* Muscle is a metabolically active tissue. Far more active than fat tissue, and, as such, it requires a precise number of calories daily to maintain itself. Therefore, the more muscle you have, the higher your BMR. This equals far more calories/fat burned (24/7), even while your body is at rest. (Ladies, this is why men can lose weight so much quicker. But don't be discouraged. Put down the latte, grab the weights—and watch your body change.)

▶ It takes about 20 minutes of moderate to intense aerobic (not anaerobic) exercise before your body will shift from burning glycogen to a slower burning, more efficient fuel. That fuel being stored body fat, i.e., free fatty acids.

▶ Eat sugar, crave sugar. Eat sugar, wear it as fat. Eat sugar, be moody, anxious, depressed, and with low, sporadic energy levels. Eat sugar, increase your risks for perpetual health conditions.

▶ For those who don't care about a lean, attractive body, I must ask: *"How you do feel about cancer?"* As reported by the American Cancer Society: *"Being overweight can increase your risk of cancer by 50%."* Overweight men had significantly higher mortality ratios for prostate cancer, while overweight women had significantly higher rates for ovarian and breast cancer.)

▶ Protein and fat build and repair the body. Carbohydrates do not.

▶ Healthy fats are a must for the brain and body to thrive.

▶ Carbs need to be used as energy, or they'll be headed to fat storage. Whereas with protein and healthy dietary fat, the body can utilize an excess of these nutrients for rebuilding the body's cells, hormones, muscle, neurotransmitters, etc.

▶ The most effective method to lose body fat, and keep it off longterm, is to build LBM, eat plenty of healthy fat, quality protein, minimal carbs, and maintain your serotonin.

▶ Buy organic, fresh food, not processed. Pre-packaged/processed food has so many harmful ingredients added. Plus, they cost more. Example: Ready-to-cook turkey patties with goat cheese. Healthy, right? Nope. Read the ingredient panel. Numerous chemicals, sweeteners, etc., added to this otherwise healthy food.

▶ Maintaining healthy levels of serotonin = controlling carb cravings and binge eating, reducing body fat, water retention, depression, anxiety, panic attacks, alleviating mood swings, aggression, SAD, ADD, ADHD, OCD, PMS, suicidal behavior, migraines, chronic pain disorders, while improving sleep patterns, heart health, libido, etc.

▶ For those individuals who smoke, take drugs (prescription, OTC, or recreational), eat sugar, processed/refined food, drink alcohol, caffeine, sodas, consume HFCS, corn syrup, aspartame, neotame, sucralose, and other artificial sweeteners, eat a low fat/fat-free diet, along with living a sedentary lifestyle—and yet don't have a weight or health problem, BEWARE. Don't let this fool you. The serious health risks associated with living such an unhealthy lifestyle can literally take years to surface. Damage is indeed being done at the cellular level and you will, sooner or later, reap what you sow.

▶ If you want to live a long, happy, and healthy life, you must live a healthy lifestyle. This healthy lifestyle is, though, completely dependent upon you being able to properly maintain your serotonin.

▶ To help ensure you achieve and maintain healthy levels of this major neurotransmitter, find a quality 5-HTP and take it faithfully every day. (I use NOW brand.)

▶ Maintaining your serotonin will, undoubtedly, help you live this much-needed healthier lifestyle. But you must also be <u>willing</u> to make the effort to break old unhealthy habits, and you must exercise weekly, preferably weight training. Please do not wait until you're sick, suffering with heart disease, diabetes, cancer, or on your death bed, before you decide to live this healthier lifestyle. Please make the effort starting today for you, and those you love. This is your L-I-F-E. What will you do with it? Please, don't procrastinate another moment. You can do this. I promise. Define—*and defy your age.*

Body by Phoenix Client Testimonials

"At age 51, I was rapidly heading down the slippery menopausal slope. Diet and exercise didn't stop the weight gain or expanding waistline. Then I met Phoenix and she changed my life. As my trainer and nutrition expert for the next 3 years, she totally changed my body with her results-oriented methods. Now, at 59, having moved to another state, I no longer have Phoenix to work with, but I have the foundation she gave me to keep me on track. I enjoy an active, prescription drug-free life. I wear a size 4—and feel better now than I did at age 40. Thank you, Phoenix!!"

— Sherry Kennedy, 59, Wife, Mother, Grandmother, Retired CFO

"Phoenix says to 'define your age!' Thanks to her, I'm 67 and getting younger! I can't say enough good things about Phoenix. I've been working with her for almost 7 years. During that time, I've lost 40 pounds and gone from a size 16 to a 4. Phoenix has done the research, and her advice is spot on! I'm proof that it works! Without her, we would NEVER get to where we are! I'm retired and able to enjoy life, thanks in large part to her! If I can do this, anyone can. Thank you, Phoenix, for giving me the health, energy, and time, so as to enjoy my grandkids!"

— Nancy Loeffel, 67, Wife, Mother, Grandmother, Retired Educator

"When I met Phoenix, I had no idea how much my life would change and all for the better! I was struggling with insomnia, depression, poor eating, weight gain, and with no direction on how to fix this mess called my 'body.' Phoenix taught me how to read labels, how to eat, when to eat, serotonin's role, healthy fat, and much more. Every day, through tough love and compassion, Phoenix challenges me to be better, live healthier, be leaner, be stronger, be kinder, push harder, be an aware consumer, seek healthier options, which all makes a more beautiful, healthier and happier ME!!!!"

— Raechelle Chisolm, 41, Mother, Business Woman

"I'm so thankful to have found Phoenix. Her passion for helping people has inspired and motivated me to become lean and healthy. Her guidance has changed my life! I will forever be grateful!"

— Mary Angell Harmon, 45, Wife, Mother, Educator

"It gives me pleasure to share my transformation, from a 66 year old woman who, unfortunately, accepted what our culture expects a woman of my age to accept—to a 69 year old woman who feels and looks better than ever! Phoenix's passion is contagious, resulting in a wonderful partnership. She's taught me how to eat so I can be lean and healthy; including body, mind, and soul. I no longer crave the wine or carbs I used to love. My life has changed in so many ways, resulting in peace about my age and excitement about my future. Thus, giving me confidence in my strength, as a woman, mother, grandmother and wife."

— Connie Morrow, 69, Wife, Mother, Grandmother

"I walked into Phoenix's studio wearing a size 22, 217 lbs, nearly 44% body fat, and feeling terrible about myself. In our time together, I learned about serotonin, how to read food labels, and how to lose weight by eating the right food. I also learned how to control my cravings. I lost 75 lbs and 13.8% body fat. I now wear a size 8. But my transformation was more than physical. My life no longer revolves around food. I have also made myself a priority. I feel great! Phoenix is a great partner who is passionate about helping her clients exceed their goals. I can't thank her enough!"

— Cami Legacy, 53, Wife, Mother, Senior HR Consultant Wellstar Hospital

"Phoenix, thank you for teaching me what you call, 'The Science of Nutrition,' along with the crucial role of serotonin. You have freed me from the nutritional mistakes that prevented me from regaining control of my health. Your book, nutritional expertise, and excellent training, have equipped me with the skills and confidence to rewrite a healthier future for myself and my family."

— LaShanda Gordon, 44, Wife, Mother, Regulatory Medical Writer

"Working with Phoenix is a game changer! I was an overweight, pre-diabetic, busy mom with no hope for change. Phoenix's expertise as a nutritionist, trainer, and her knowledge about serotonin, led me to a healthy A1c, and a stronger, much leaner body with a totally different mindset. She helped me make a transformation inside, that created a beautiful transformation on the outside."

— Denise Cisel Meier, 47, business owner, wife, mother

"I've been the queen of yo-yo dieting all my life. Not until I found Phoenix, who is a fabulous trainer and expert nutritionist, did I finally understand how both work together to achieve maximum health. I learn everyday from her, while getting stronger, physically and mentally. I feel fabulous!"

— Jane Goff, 51, Retired Educator

"Phoenix has truly transformed my health in just six short months. I'm stronger, leaner, and my daily anxiety is gone, because of her training, guidance on nutrition, and teaching me all about the 5 and serotonin. Phoenix is a joy to work with and I am thankful I found her!"

— Shelley Looper, 47, wife, mother

"Phoenix's training and nutritional advice is second to none. She brings decades of knowledge and expertise. She inspires, motivates, challenges, educates....Phoenix gets results!"

— Tiffany Tabb, 45, Wife, Mother, Realtor

"Phoenix is a master alchemist who mixes solid scientific research, nutrition, targeted exercise, and a whole lot of compassion to conjure up magical transformations in her clients. Before I began working with Phoenix, I had (almost) passively accepted that sluggishness and creeping weight gain were natural consequences of aging. But Phoenix has helped renew my vitality, health, and outlook—with the added bonus of significant weight loss. At age 58, I'm leaner and more energetic than I've been in years."

— Melinda J. Matthews, 58, Wife, Mother, Writer, Editor

"Phoenix is a kind, caring lifesaver. When I started with her, I was physically sick every day depressed, and overweight. Now, at the age of 51, I've never felt better and I owe it all to Phoenix's dedication to me and my health! Thanks for all you have done for me!!"

— Marla Garrett, 52, Business Owner

"In only a few months, Phoenix helped me make extraordinary changes, losing weight and weaning me off an antidepressant, was just the beginning. I've never felt better, or more hopeful. And Phoenix never gives up on me, no matter my struggles."

— Kathie Gerber, 62, Wife, Mother, Business Woman

RESEARCH/REFERENCES

<u>Books/Health References:</u>
5-HTP, The Natural Way to Overcome Depression, Obesity, and Insomnia, Michael T. Murray, ND

The Schwarzbein Principle, Diana Schwarzbein, MD and Nancy Deville

Psychiatry—The Ultimate Fraud, Bruce Wiseman

The Cholesterol Myths, Uffe Ravnskov, MD, PhD

Grain Brain, Dr. David Perlmutter

Good Calories, Bad Calories, Gary Taubes

Ageless: The Naked Truth About Bioidentical Hormones, Suzanne Somers

Calculated Risks: How to Know When Numbers Deceive You, Gerd Gigerenzer

The Food Revolution: How Your Diet Can Help Save Your Life and Our World, John Robbins

Natural Cures "They" Don't Want You to Know About, Kevin Trudeau

The Shooting Drugs; Prozac and It's Generation Exposed, Donna Smart

Solving the Depression Puzzle, Rita Elkins, MH

The Glucose Revolution, Jennie Miller, PhD; Thomas Wolever, MD, PhD; Stephen Colagiuri, MD; Kaye Powell, M. Nutr., Dietician

Prescription for Nutritional Healing, Phyllis Balch, CNC; James Balch, MD

Natural Hormone Balance for Women, Uzzi Reiss, MD, OB/GYN

Never an Outbreak, William Fharel

<u>Research/Clinical Support:</u>
Wurtman and Wurtman, "Brain serotonin carbohydrate cravings, obesity, and depression." *Advances in Experimental Medicine and Biology* 398 (1996)

Poldinger W, et al. A functional-dimensional approach to depression: serotonin deficiency as a target syndrome in a comparison of 5-HTP and fluvoxamine. Psychopathology 1991;24:53-81.

Cangiano C, et al. Eating behavior and adherence to dietary prescriptions in obese adult subjects treated with 5-hydroxytryptophan. Am J Clin Nutr 1992;56:863-7.

Zmilacher K, et al. L-5-hydroxytryptophan alone and in combination with a peripheral decarboxylase inhibitor in the treatment of depression. Neuropsychobiology 1988;20:28-35.

Van Praag H. Management of depression with serotonin precursors. Biol Psychiatry 1981;16:291-310. Byerley W, et al. 5-hydroxytryptophan: a review of its antidepressant efficacy and adverse effects. J Clin Psychopharmacol 1987;7:127.

Maissen CP, et al. Comparison of the effect of 5-hydroxytryptophan and propranolol in the interval treatment of migraine. Schweiz Med Wochenschr 1991;121:1585-90

J.E. Blundel and M.B. Leshem, "The effect of 5-HTP on food intake and on the anorexic action of amphetamine and fenfluramine," *Journal of Pharmacy and Pharmacology* 27 (1975) 31-37

F. Ceci, "The effects of oral 5-HTP administration on feeding behavior in obese adult female patients." *Journal of Neural Transmission* 76 (1989) 109-17

Wurtman and Wurtman, *The Serotonin Solution*, and *Nutrition and the Brain*

H. M. Van Praag, "Management of depression with serotonin precursors." *Biological Psychiatry* 16, (1981) 290-311.

J.J. Alino, J.L. Gutierrez, and M. Iglesias, "5-HTP and an MAOI in the treatment of depression. A double-blind study," *International Pharmacopsychiatry* 11 (1976) 8-15

Benket, "Effect of parachlorophenylalnine and 5-HTP on human sexual behavior." *Monographs in Neural Sciences* 3 (1976) 88-93

R.J. Wyatt, "Effects of 5-HTP on the sleep of normal human subjects." *Electroencephalography and Clinical Neurophysiology* 30 (1971) 505-10

Research in Depression, Advances in Biochemical Psychopharmacology, Vol. 39, pg. 301-313

Gastpar and Wakelin (1988), Selective 5-HTP Reuptake Inhibitors: *Novel or Commonplace Agents?* Advances in Biological Psychiatry Vol. 19 pg. 18-30 and 52-57

Schwarcz, Young, and Brown (1989), Kynurenine and Seretonin Pathways Progress in Trytophan research Advances in Experimental Medicine and Biology, Vol. 29

<u>Websites</u>:
PETA: peta.com/Viva! USA: vivausa.org
Meet Your Meat: meetyourmeat.com
realhealth@healthiernews.com
cchrint.org/2009/08/12/the-prozac-calamity
Centers for Disease Control and Prevention: cdc.gov
National Institutes of Health: nih.gov
nutritiondata.com/index.html
mercola.com/article/statins.htm
thenutritionreporter.com/fructose_dangers.html
usatoday.com/news/health/2004-03-25-hfcs-usat_x.htm
cspinet.org/sodapop/liquid_candy.htm
upliftprogram.com/depression_stats.html
niddk.nih.gov/health/nutrit/pubs/unders.htm
medical-library.net/sites/framer.html?/sites/_adult_onset_diabetes
4.dr-rath-foundation.org/PHARMACEUTICAL_BUSINESS/laws_of_the_pharmaceutical_industry.htm
muscletech.com/CALCULATORS/PROTEIN/Protein_Calculator

In Loving Memory of

Kashif, Greta, Gunther, Ella, Raina, Bentley, Maya, Sagan & Hudson

In closing my book, a book that is dedicated to helping others live a happier and healthier life, it was important to devote this final page to some of my beloved animals. As much as my soul thrived by loving them, they selflessly gave me more love than mere words can ever express. Kashif was the first Rott I ever rescued. She died narly 40 years ago and I still miss her! Greta and Gunther were faithfully by my side for over 12 years. Though the cycle of life is never easy, all I know is that I must give back. So, I help another animal in need. I rescued beautiful Ella, followed by adopting sweet Raina. Then I rescued helpless and oooh so neglected little Bentley. I adopted Maya and then Sagan. I rescued Hudson shortly thereafter. He was absolutely stunning in looks—and personality! Every single one of these beautiful dogs were desperately in need of someone to save them, care for them, love them, and keep them safe. I was so grateful to be that "someone." In return, I was beyond fortunate for all the love and joy they gave me!

Knowing how much each of these sweet souls (and many more), gave to me, *knowing how each one of them helped me live a more peaceful, meaningful, happier and, subsequently, healthier life*, it is, therefore, my sincerest wish that if you have yet to discover this rare and precious bond, please consider rescuing an orphan from your local shelter. You will save a life, and they, in turn, will give your life new meaning!

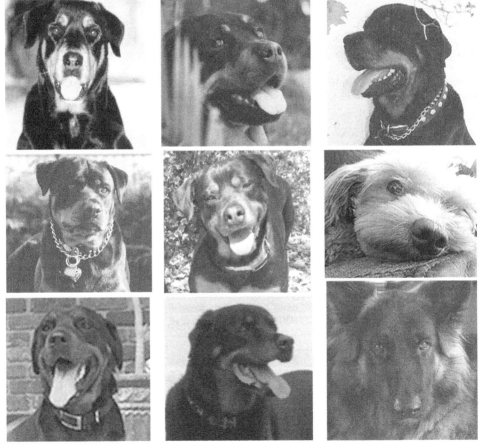

AUTHOR

If ever there was ever one so passionately motivated to make a difference, it would be, Phoenix, a truly life-changing entrepreneur. Fed up by the endless deceptions in the diet, food, and pharma' industries, she vowed to make a difference.

In addition to being an innovative trainer and nutritionist, as a respected researcher, author and weight loss/anti-aging expert, Phoenix takes her work to an entirely different level of accomplishment. Clinically supported, her research focused on neurochemistry and nutrition. By understanding how to effectively implement the science, she helps reverse and prevent various diseases, i.e., obesity, diabetes, depression, anxiety, insomnia, ADD/ADHD, PMS, hypertension, significantly lowers inflammation, body fat and triglycerides, alleviates "high cholesterol" concerns, mitigates addictions (carbs/sugar, alcohol, nicotine, and caffeine), stops a transfer of addictions, and reduces risks for heart disease, stroke, heart attack, and certain cancers.

After watching the video showcasing her work found on her website, bodybyphoenix.com, it is undeniable: Phoenix is making a difference. At 62 years young, the legitimacy of her research is also apparent in her own health and striking physique.

Phoenix's next professional endeavor? A docu-series? Host her own national talk radio show? Both would be based on her research. Both could help change even more lives. Considering our current healthcare crisis, more so, since COVID, we sincerely hope Phoenix achieves her goals.

Phoenix currently lives in the Atlanta area. She owns/operates, Body by Phoenix, a private weight loss and personal training studio. She also continues to consult with people around the world. Should you seek Phoenix's expertise, please email her at phoenix@bodybyphoenix.com.

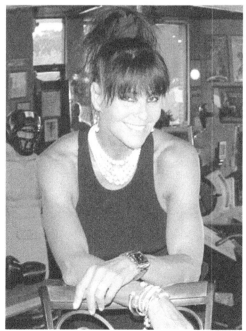

Made in the USA
Monee, IL
09 February 2024

53206835R00134